Pranayama

The Breathing Techniques for Balance Healing

(Master the Art of Pranayama Breathing and the Ujjayi Breath)

Willie Fabrizio

Published By **Simon Dough**

Willie Fabrizio

Pranayama: The Breathing Techniques for Balance Healing (Master the Art of Pranayama Breathing and the Ujjayi Breath)

ISBN   978-1-77485-486-0

No part of this guidebook shall be reproduced in any form without permission in writing from the publisher except in the case of brief quotations embodied in critical articles or reviews.

Legal & Disclaimer

The information contained in this ebook is not designed to replace or take the place of any form of medicine or professional medical advice. The information in this ebook has been provided for educational & entertainment purposes only.

The information contained in this book has been compiled from sources deemed reliable, and it is accurate to the best of the Author's knowledge; however, the Author cannot guarantee its accuracy and validity and cannot be held liable for any errors or omissions. Changes are periodically made to this book. You must consult your doctor or get professional medical advice before using any of the suggested remedies, techniques, or information in this book.

Upon using the information contained in this book, you agree to hold harmless the Author from and against any damages, costs, and expenses, including any legal fees potentially resulting from the application of any of the information provided by this guide. This disclaimer applies to any damages or injury caused by the use and application, whether directly or indirectly, of any advice or information presented, whether for breach of contract, tort, negligence, personal injury, criminal intent, or under any other cause of action.

You agree to accept all risks of using the information presented inside this book. You need to consult a professional medical practitioner in order to ensure you are both able and healthy enough to participate in this program.

TABLE OF CONTENTS

Introduction

If you've ever attended classes in yoga, meditation, or hatha and hatha yoga, you've probably seen the term "pranayama" used. If you've taken classes that have "updated" its syllabus to appear less alien in an American audience and they've likely changed the word "pranayama" with terms such as "breath control,"" "pranic breathing,"" "energy expansion" or another similar expression.

However it's generally the identical thing. Prana, as the name suggests is the Sanskrit word that means "breath" also known as "life force" however, it could also refer to "vital power," in addition to "spirit." Ayama means "to extend" or "to draw out," though it can also refer to "restraint," "control," or "stopping," in some situations.

According to ancient Indian texts there are both spiritual and psychic benefits of controlling your breath but we won't get into it here. These same texts also assert that there are emotional, mental and physical rewards for pranayama practitioners. What do you think? There's an increasing body of medical evidence that backs certain assertions.

The connection between breathing with the autonomic nervous system for a long time been recognized by doctors. This is the same for breath's connection to digestion breathing, heart rate, respiration sexual arousal, brain function and many more.

Without going into too much detail Medical researchers are now recognizing that certain breathing techniques can have tangible, extremely precise and highly reproducible effects on body and mind. This is a good thing, due to the health benefits that have been claimed by practitioners of yoga and meditation for many years are now being verified by the latest research.

It also shows that the dangers the older practitioners and writers have warned us about are real. Although pranayama is taught in a face-to-face setting by a skilled and certified instructor to prevent problems like this However, the risks that are involved are not common. The most common problems arise when practitioners attempt to push beyond their limits and disregard their body's warning signs. This guide will focus on only the things you can safely perform yourself.

Pranayama is often practiced along with the martial arts, hatha yoga and meditation. However, it is also able to be practiced on its own due to of its numerous benefits, among them, discussed in this article.

Chapter 1: A Few Words Of Caution

There are more yoga and meditation instructors in America than in India. Although this indicates that the discipline is drawing more people who are interested in it (which is great) but it is also a sign that not all of them are skilled or experienced enough to teach the practice (which is a problem).

With the number of yoga and meditation classes in America that produce instructors as if they were industrial factory products the quality of many teachers are highly doubtful. They are often featured to radio, television and various other media forms, proclaiming the benefits of hatha yoga as well as pranayama.

While these practices definitely have medical benefits that have been proven However, they do come with dangers. However, these risks are usually ignored or not even discussed in any way. This kind of ignorance or deliberate obfuscation is reckless and dangerous.

Professor Holger Cramer from The University of Duisburg Essen, Germany was the lead researcher in a study of certain risks. In "Adverse events that are associated with Yoga and Yoga: A Systematic Review of Publication Case Reports and Case Series," Cramer found that some of the most advanced types of pranayama may result in hemorrhage (swelling of blood clotted inside tissue) or pneumothorax (air or gas that is absorbed by the lung's cavity as well as in the chest's wall and causes the lungs to shrink).

in the February 2007 issue of the Emergency Journal, A.S. Kashyap, K.P. Anand along with S. Kashyap, published an article titled "Complications of Yoga." In the report, they assert it was they believe that the Valsalva Maneuver was responsible for the occurrence of some cases of subcutaneous Emphysema (when air is accumulated within pockets under the skin or in the abdomen).

There's a huge amount of Sanskrit texts that contain these warnings, however they are not known to the majority of teachers who are widely distributed. If you are in one of the classes where the instructor states that there is no risk involved with doing pranayama, you should you should leave the class immediately and seek the money back.

Be aware that your body is equipped with its own internal system of wisdom and warnings and you must be aware of it. If you notice any discomfort, such as nausea, dizziness headaches, shortness or breath or blurred vision it is best to stop right away and report it to the doctor. Perhaps even contact your doctor.

It's not easy to build strength and stamina in a day. The fit ones started slow, building the body over time, and with a lot of patience and perseverance. Similar is the case with pranayama. The benefits are evident however, you must be patient, consistent and slow down a bit - whatever your gym's yoga instructor may suggest.

Chapter 2: Dos And Don'ts To Consider When Practicing Pranayama

It is best to practice pranayama outdoors and in the countryside, where the air is healthy and healthy. It's obvious that this isn't feasible for everyone, particularly those who live in crowded cities.

If you're required to take it indoors, select an area that's clean, free of damp, mold and dust in addition, one that offers excellent ventilation. A room that's newly painted isn't a good option for many reasons even if you keep doors open.

Don't perform pranayama after eating. When you practice it on an empty stomach could cause digestive problems like diarrhea, constipation, bloating or lethargy and abdominal discomforts. It is best to wait at the minimum two hours following a meal before practicing pranayama, however, it's also contingent upon your mood. If you still feel hungry after 3 hours you should wait a bit longer.

Although there are various types of pranayama that could be performed to alleviate thirst and hunger but it is best to practice them only after you've learned the basics. We'll go over them in the last section. If you're hungry take a bite of food and put off eating for at least 2 hours prior to doing pranayama. If you're taking small bites of food, such as a banana it's enough to wait for one hour.

Every exercise should be conducted using empty bowels and bladders. Be sure to reserve enough time to do this exercise. If you're stressed it's easy to do the routine in order to get it done and then it becomes useless.

If you're suffering from breathing problems (such like asthma) you should talk to your primary physician regarding what you can and cannot do, and the length of time you can stay. Concerning expecting mothers, it's recommended to seek advice from an expert. Medically-certified and certified yoga instructors that are trained specifically for expecting mothers, therefore you may consider looking them up.

People suffering from colds, coughs and severe constipation should avoid sittingkari pranayama. Sitali pranayama is forbidden for those suffering from coughs, colds, or tonsillitis. If you suffer from excessive blood pressure stay clear of the bhastrika and surya bedhana pranayama. It is not advised for those suffering from heart ailments and ulcers.

If you suffer from an abnormally low blood pressure you shouldn't practice ujjayi pranayama. In some instances, ujjayi is also not advised for people suffering from heart or hypertension. People with ear issues (such as otitis media, glue ears as well as swimmer's ear) are advised to stay clear of the bhramari pranayama.

Sometimes even after consulting with an expert or your doctor there is a chance that you will experience discomfort, especially at the beginning of your journey out. If you are worried about being repetitive, keep in mind that your body is a source of own wisdom, which you must listen to and follow.

Chapter 3: Preparation Before The Beginning

In all other instances, except for hatha yoga pranayama is to be performed standing straight with your back straight, and your jaw straight with the floor. If you tilt your head back or backwards or slouching your shoulders back or forward, can hinder the flow air through your stomach or your throat and cause nausea or dizziness.

Sit properly

While maintaining a straight and upright posture, it is important to take as much time as you can to relax. Although it might seem like an ideal idea to choose an ergonomic chair that has a back rest, it's not. Certain back supports cause users to lean forward and others make you lean backwards. Others keep you standing, but the seat's angle creates pressure that is uncomfortable on your buttocks and spine.

Yoga practitioners typically lie across the floor with their feet together but we're not practicing Hatha yoga here. If you're more comfortable somewhere other that the ground, opt for the backless or stool chair. Avoid the deep cushions that take you over. You need a cushion that allows you to sit up straight as well as assist to keep that posture for at minimum five minutes.

Relax

Tensify your feet, craning them into a ball and remain in this position for a long time, counting slowly to three. After that, let them go. Relax and enjoy the feeling that your feet should radiate.

Repeat the exercise by putting your calves first, the upper legs next, followed by your thighs, and finally your stomach, followed by your chest, followed by your hands and arms followed by your neck jaw and your face. Make sure you spend minimum three seconds tensing each body part, and then spend for a few minutes, enjoy the feeling of relaxation before moving on to the next part of your body.

Although you don't need to practice this every time you go for an hour, this kind of relaxing, relaxed feeling is what your whole body should feel before you start.

Breathe properly

The majority of pranayama exercises are performed using the nose, and seldom using the mouth. Furthermore, nearly all exercises require breathing through your abdomen, which is known as belly breathing. However, in certain situations the breath be absorbed into the chest. Therefore, you must learn to separate your breathing correctly.

Unless stated otherwise Keep your lips shut and your jaw in a relaxed position. If you're performing the second properly, there should be gaps between your lower and upper teeth. The tongue's tip should be also pressed against the sides of your upper teeth.

Chapter 4: Adham Pranayama (Abdominal Breath)

If you observe children and toddlers, they breathe in their stomachs naturally this is a process known as diaphragmatic breathing or abdominal breathing. Later on, we will begin breath through the chests, referred to as collarbone breathing or clavicular breathing. The latter is not good for health since it limits our oxygen consumption and doesn't adequately let out toxic substances.

Adham pranayama is the most common exercise, so only proceed with the other exercises after you've completed the exercise. You should sit in the mirror (not essential). Exhale and spread your fingers and place them on your stomachs and make sure that your middle fingers are touching the belly button. Inhale and take your breath straight into your stomach , while maintaining your chest in a relaxed position.

If you've done this correctly the fingers should be spread widely and the points of the middle finger should slide apart and your shoulders should not be raised (if you're unable to tell take yourself before the mirror). If your shoulders do raise and you're breathing through your chest, and you haven't isolated your abdomen properly. Imagine your in-breath being the method used to blast your stomach up like balloons. Consider your out-breath like pulling your stomach back into your spine.

Begin each breath with an incredibly slow count of three at a time. When your breath in, you should think, "one one thousand, two one thousand three one thousand" and then repeat the counting while you exhale. Beginning with the number three is suggested. As you become familiar with the method you can gradually up the number to 10 but be careful not to push it too far. Only do what you are at ease with.

Another variation is to breathe directly into your stomach to get a fixed count, then hold the breath to a set count, then exhale to the same number of times. After a one-second breath pause, breathe in again. Another variation is to breathe in and breathe, then exhale and after which you hold your breath in the same order. If you're starting with a count of 3 such as: inhale for three times and breathe for three times and exhale for 3 counts and then take your time and hold the breath until three times.

Clavicular breathing is beneficial when you're active, but when you're not active, it can result in stress. According to the traditional Indian medical practices (called the ayurveda) it could cause digestive issues constipation, digestive upsets, as well as other gynaecological issues. Your diaphragm acts as an additional heart. Breathing through your abdomen allows it to draw in more blood venous, which increases circulation throughout the body.

It is recommended to do this for approximately 5 minutes in the morning before breakfast and in the evening prior to dinner. It not only relaxes and helps you focus, but it can also help reduce anxiety and tension, headaches and pain in the menstrual cycle.

Chapter 5: Nadhi Sodhana Pranayama (Alternate Nostril Breath)

According to Sanskrit texts Alternate nostril breathing regulates nerves, concentrates the mind and enhances concentration. Prior to any meditation or prayer it is therefore recommended to do this pranayama. is often recommended to provide "oomph" when you are asking God for something. Ayurveda suggests this practice is believed to combat colds, regulate the body's temperature, and boost the respiratory and circulatory systems.

A study carried out by the Tagore Medical College & Hospital in India appears to support the idea. Researchers under the direction of Dr. D.V. Sivapriya discovered that it could help improve the lung function. Their research paper, released in the 2010 edition of the journal Recent Research in Science and Technology and Technology, claims that those who performed this practice over a period of 45 days demonstrated enhanced cognitive capabilities.

The exercise is also known as aniloma-viloma, which Ayurvedic doctors recommend to treat lethargy and gout, excess fat and mucus. The article also states that this practice can ensure regular bowel movements as well as reduce the effects of the effects of sleep and eating problems.

Make sure you hold the right side of your hand (or your left hand, in case you're more comfortable with it) and put your thumb on your nostril on the left. Set your index finger in front of the nose (at the point between your eyebrows) to help balance your hands. The middle of your finger must be resting against the left nostril.

Exhale and let your abdomen empty of air. Connect your right nostril using your thumb, and plug your left nostril using the middle of your finger. It is not necessary to press your nostrils down instead, but you should you can plug them by squeezing your middle finger and your thumb in a gentle manner by putting your nose between them.

Unplug your left nose and breathe it in for three slow counts. Connect it again and exhale from your right nostril to a slow count of three. Next, breathe in using the left nostril to count slowly three. Exhale from your left nostril to an extended counting of 3. This is a complete cycle of nadi.

Another variation is the use of jalandhara bandha (throat lock). Remove the left nostril plug and breathe in, then connect it and breathe in. Unplug your right nostril , and breathe it out and then breathe into it. Plug it in and breathe deeply. Inhale using the left side of your nose. This is also a complete Nadhi Sodhana cycle.

The time spent inhaling and taking your breath in, and then exhaling, must be the same. If you take just three minutes inhaling you must be able to keep your breath in for three seconds, then exhale for 3 seconds. After each exhalation, there needs to be at least a 1 second space before you breathe in, again.

WARNING!

Certain forms of pranayama that are more advanced will require you at exhaling air while maintaining your throat and nose closed. This is how people try to alleviate stress on their ears while they descend from a high altitude. Doctors refer to this as the Valsalva procedure, which is associated with serious medical dangers, and should be kept away from.

If you practice nadi sadhana with the jalandhara variation it is important to keep your breath. Do not try to expel the air and keep your throat and nasal passages closed.

Another alternative is to keep your breath in between having completed the cycle. It is when you exhale out of one nostril on your left, plug it in, take your breath in for exact same time and then disconnect your left nostril, and then inhale to start your next cycle. This is recommended especially for menstrual cramps and stomach upsets.

In Ayurveda, if feel like you're breathing through just one nostril despite breathing through your nose you're probably heading to an acute cold or fever. The pranayama practice can help ease this, however ayurveda suggests slowing down your pace and eating well in addition to drinking plenty of fluids.

Chapter 6: Surya And Chandra Bedhana Pranayama (Sun And Moon Breaths That Pierce)

Left or right nostril breathing is a variation of the nadhi sodhana. In ayurveda and hatha yoga one nostril on the right is believed to be associated to the sun (surya) and therefore is believed to be a source of warmth. The left nostril on the contrary, is linked with moon (chandra) it is also believed to increase cooling.

SURYA BEDHANA PRANAYAMA

In your left nostril, plug it the same way as you do with Nadhi Sodhana. Inhale and exhale through the right nostril and repeat until you reach three. Another option could be to inhale and hold your breath for a few seconds, then exhale using only your right nostril.

As this increases temperatures in the body, this practice can be used to combat the symptoms of sluggishness, fatigue, colds as well as prior to engaging in any demanding physical exercise. If you've had abdominal or heart, brain, or surgery should consult with their GPs prior to performing this. People who suffer from high blood pressure ought to be avoiding this completely.

CHANDRA BEDHANA PRANAYAMA

This is exactly the opposite of surya pranayama bedhana, in which you breathe through only the left nostril. There is no evidence of contraindications to this practice that is utilized to treat anxiety, fever hypertension, and premature ejaculation. Chandra bedhana pranayama can be recommended for people who exhibit temperament or people who are stressed about things.

Note:

Right and left nostril breathing fall under tradition of folk remedies across India, Nepal, Assam as well as Bhutan since the remedies are prescribed by ayurvedic practitioners. Therefore, they are viewed only as treatments, not general cures.

A consistent daily practice of Nadhi Sodhana, in conjunction with a balanced eating plan, consistent exercise and enough rest, is believed to alleviate the majority of illnesses. If you notice that you have recourse to surya bedhana and the chandra bedhana routinely that indicates (to the Ayurvedic brain) that there is an imbalance in your body . You should consult an expert.

Chapter 7: Ujjayi Pranayama (Victorious Or Conquering Breath)

It's a little tricky without someone else to guide the way, so let's do this step slowly. In order to do this, you'll need to restrict your throat to ensure that your in-breath as well as out-breath sounds can be heard. One way to begin is to lower your chin slightly. This will create a small obstruction to the airway just below your collarbone. It will feel tight.

Another method to create the effect you want is use your thumb and put it with care inside the throat's hollow near your collarbone. If you feel like you're choked then you're pushing too hard. Back off a bit. Then breathe. If you're breathing correctly your out-breath as well as in-breath will produce a wheezing sound. It's as if there is the throat mucus.

Try to use the word "aah," while sucking your breath into. The majority of us are used to making sounds only when the exhale. However, not when we inhale. Inhaling and making a sound can cause you to be aware of what's happening in your throat, specifically when you use your glottis.

The glottis, or glottis, is the area of the throat that is constricted to produce the H K the G (as the case with "Grover," not "George") as well as Ng sounds. You should constrict your throat so that you create the sound of the H when you breathe out and in while keeping your lips shut.

You're not trying to make a growl or Darth Vader type sound. If tightening your throat makes it itchy or makes you cough or causes your breath to be hear by someone in the room, you've tense your throat too much. If you're doing the right thing it's only you (and the person sitting next to you) will be able to be able to hear what "ocean noise" (as the yogis refer to it) your breathing produces.

Find the perfect level of tension that permits you to make this sound without discomfort at all and to keep it for a long time. Once you've found the perfect level of tension and you're now ready to start.

Maintain your straight posture with your jaw being parallel to the floor. You should be looking directly ahead (though you may also close the eyes). Make sure you tighten your glottis to ensure that you create an "ocean sounds." In ujjayi practice, you breathe in and out but you don't hold the breath indefinitely. Be sure to make sure you have a consistent volume "ocean sounds" is uniform as well as that your out-breath and in-breath are identical length. One exhalation and one breath is considered to be one cycle.

Ujjayi is the initial step in a journey to deep meditation. It can help increase the body's heat, improving oxygenation of blood, controlling blood pressure and clearing out toxins in the body. It is also suggested for people suffering from insomnia and menstrual cramps.

Chapter 8: Kapalbhati And Bhastrika Pranayama (Shining Skull And Bellows Breath)

Many teachers use the two terms in a way that is wrong. Both pranayamas should not be practiced by pregnant women and those suffering from hypertension, high blood pressure and heart disease, hernia and ulcers.

KAPALBHATI PRANAYAMA

Kapal is not just a reference to the skull, but also to everything connected to itincluding the brain, the organs inside as well as the exterior of the face. It is believed to treat the cranial sinuses, anemia and cranial sinuses and also to cleanse the respiratory system as well as aid in weight loss. Bhati refers to the way it firms up the skin and gives it a shine, which is the result of an increase in oxygen levels to blood. Kapalbhati claims to protect beauty and rejuvenates.

This is a recommended practice for those who smoke, since it is believed that it cleanses the lung. It also helps strengthen the abdominal muscles, people who have trouble digesting and irregular stool movements should practice it frequently. Many studies show that it's also beneficial for those suffering from asthma and bronchitis however, it is recommended to consult your GP before attempting this.

In kapalbhati breathing, you breathe the same way as you do in ujjayi However, the focus is on exhalation. Instead of a soft out-breath however, you should pull your abdomen swiftly and sharply into your spine. This will trigger several loud exhalations via your nostrils (NOT your mouth!). Exhalations should be non-sensical that result from an exhalation action that is triggered after you have pushed your breath out (again by using your nose).

Inhalation with recoil of one exhalation every second is a good speed, however, two exhalations every second is considered the best but going slower is thought to be ineffective. However, you should select the pace that you feel comfortable with. Begin with a steady flow for a minute, and then stop and re-start the exercise. You can increase the duration as you become better and more powerful.

BHASTRIKA PRANAYAMA

Imagine how ironsmiths pump their bellows quickly and rhythmically to keep a temperature high within his forge. This is the reason it's also known as"agni pranayama" (fire breathing). You should only do this when you're familiar with kapalbhati.

In this version it is a similar importance given to exhaling as well. This should also be performed with Ujjayi. The length and quantity of your in-breath should be the same as the volume of your out-breath. Between each exhalation or inhalation it is recommended to take an instant break. A one-inhalation-pause and an exhalation pause is a complete cycle. A good cycle should last for about a second, and two cycles in a second is considered to be good.

Chapter 9: Bhramari Pranayama (Humming Bee Breath)

This is a good option to improve the strength of the nerve system. It is also recommended for increasing energy levels, increasing the flow of nutrients into cells, easing migraines and headaches and also decreasing blood pressure. For those who suffer from poor short-term memory loss and lack of concentration are also advised to practice this practice.

Recent research suggests that this practice could help treat certain forms of obsessive-compulsive disorder. Others have also found that it may help regulate the endocrinal system which is beneficial for women who are pregnant. If you spend a lot of time watching a screen it is possible that you will benefit from this.

Bhramari uses the shanmukhi mudra, which is a hand gesture that you place on your face. Let's begin by examining the first issue. The mask is also known for its closing seven gates: two ears, the two eyes, two nostrils and the mouth.

Make sure you use your thumbs to press against your tragi. The tragus is a hard area of your ear, which is linked to the cheek. It's located above the ear lobe , and it is a bit higher than the ear hole. By pressing your thumbs against your tragi won't stop the sound, but it is recommended to apply pressure but with enough gentleness to block out the sound.

Close your eyes and gently place the index fingers of your lids closed so that your fingers rest on your eyes, while your tips rest on the space between your eyes and the top bridge of your nose. If you notice streaks or colors If you see colors or spots, you're pressing too hard.

The middle fingers' tips should rest on the opposite the side of your nose, about halfway between the point of the index fingers are as well as your nose. Your ring fingers must rest on the other the side of your nose but don't close them as you would do with Nadhi Sodhana.

Your pinky fingers must rest on your lips that are closed, or underneath you lower lips in order to "seal the entrance of your mouth." To ensure that you keep it sealed, fill gaps between lower and upper teeth by gently biting them. Ayurveda is a unique variant of the meridian points that are used in acupuncture and acupressure that's why you need to do this correctly (though there are variations).

When you have your mudra in place then breathe deeply and typically through your nose (no Ujjayi) inhaling all the breath into your abdominal. Exhale and then you should make a humming sound like bees. There is no hold of breath in this case, so an inhalation that is quiet and a exhalation that is humming is considered to be one cycle. Similar to all other forms of pranayama duration of each breath in and out-breath has to be the same.

Chapter 10: Sitali And Sitkari Pranayama (Cooling And Sipping Or Hissing Breath)

In a place that is generally warm and poor as India the two are extremely popular even among non-yoga enthusiasts. They both are sure to keep your body cool, and five to ten times can help reduce thirst and hunger which makes them a favourite for weight-loss enthusiasts.

Sitali and Sitkari are also recommended as remedies for laziness, and for reducing mucus and bile, and to ease the pain of arthritis. At the time of writing however, no definitive research has been conducted on the claims made, but research into their capacity to decrease hot flashes is promising.

The pranayamas are both unique as they both require you to breathe in with your mouth.

SITALI PRANAYAMA

To do this, you'll need to create a tube out of your tongue by curving the sides and pressing them in. Take your tongue out of your mouth and then take into gas through the tube that you've made through your abdominal. There should be a small sound of hissing as you go about this. Make sure you control the sound to ensure that it's not overly harsh, rough or erratic. You want smooth and consistent sound that doesn't squeak or rumble.

After your abdomen is filled and your tongue is firmly in place, you can stick it back into your mouth, seal your lips and grind your teeth gently as you breathe. Inhale and exhale through your nostrils. In-breaths, held breaths, and out-breath must be of the same length. Together, they count as one count.

SITKARI PRANAYAMA

If you aren't able to bend your tongues into perfect tubes, rest easy. The ability to do this is genetically inherited, according to research and that's what sitkari solves. In this variant the mouth is opened and expose your teeth placing your upper teeth on top of those below. Put the end of your tongue on the top of your upper teeth the same as you do when you pronounce D L, N and T.

Breathe in with your teeth, bringing the air and bringing it down to your stomach. If you've put your tongue in the correct position there should be some slight sound when you breathe in. After your abdomen is filled then close your mouth and let your upper jaw sink into a comfortable and comfortable bite. Then, keep your breath. Then, exhale through your nostrils.

Like sitali, your inbreath, held-breath, as well as out-breath must be the same length that is why they all count.

Chapter 11: Pranayama Breathing

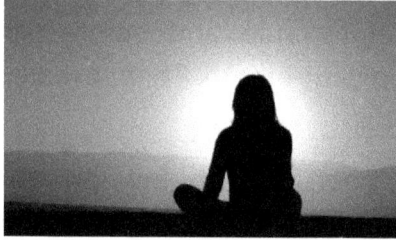

A majority of people charge their cell phones before going to bed However, how can you recharge your mind? The easiest and most effective method could be to simply focus on your breathing.

Pranayama originates from Pranayama is a Sanskrit word which refers to breathing exercises in yoga that enhance physical health, improve mental clarity, ease tension, and boost energy. The term "breathwork" can be a new word that is applied to pranayama and breathing exercises.

It is an old Indian system that defines prana as the life force or energy that is universal. force that separates people who have died from those that are living. The life force or energy is a flow of energy through channels referred to as Nadi and chakra's energy centers.

Prana is an essential energy we require in our physical and subtle layers. If we do not have it, we'll die. Prana is the reason we live.

Prana is a word with many meanings including consciousness energy, the physical breath of our bodies to our creativity, which gave birth to the kundalini shakti. Yogis will inform you that the entire universe was created out of prana.

Prana isn't easy to comprehend since we don't visualize it. However, the feeling of it is there. With a clear understanding of what prana really is and not and you will feel so connected that you are able to feel prana. When we are able to connect with prana, it will allow us to be connected to the world and discover who we really are.

Although prana is a reference to breath but it's not our actual breath. It's a form of energy that moves throughout our body via channels. It's akin with the central nervous system. These channels connect all the parts of the body and mind, and act as a conduit for prana.

Over 3000 years of in which references to prana transcends religious traditions and different cultures. Prana is a key element of tantric yoga, Ayurvedic, hatha yoga and Hindu practices, yet all of them refer to"the "life energy." It is the Hebrew word ruah and the Islamic's ruh, and the pneuma of the ancient Greeks and the anima of the ancient Romans as well as the Chinese Chi can be found in the Holy Spirit of the Christian.

Although it may not be as simple like breathing. Prana could be defined as breathing or breath. The definitions of soul include spirit the inner wind vital spiritual energy, winds, which is also known as the life force.

There are some traditions that have discovered Between five to ten prana varieties that refer to upward, downward outward and inward-moving energy, or energy that is connected to certain areas of the body such as the digestive throat, heart, or head.

Each human being has the body. Also, we have an energetic body and physical shape. Our active body can be known as"the invisible body. It's what many call an aura because it goes over the body. It is said that "they make a room glow." That's where the phrase comes from. It's how we feel the energy of someone else.

The subtle body is home to a central nervous system comprised up of nadis , or channels that are comprised by one channel as well as two additional channels which are sometimes referred to as the sun and moon and 72,000 channels. Based on the traditions it could be seventy-two channels.

Sun channel also called Pingala is located to the spine's right side. It is symbolized as "ha" which is Sanskrit. It is a channel of red in which aversions, ignorance separation, jealousy and anger thrive. They all have "hot" energies are linked to the sun.

When this energy moves across the Pingala channel when we exhale, it is possible to feel a sense of the feeling of rejection. It is possible to label ignorance in this way because we believe that eliminating certain things or individuals in our lives would result in satisfaction. However, a wise person recognizes that happiness is only found within us.

The channel of moon, also known as Ida, is located to the left side of the spine. It is symbolized in the form of "tha" as in Sanskrit. All cool energies are reflected through this channel. It is akin to ignorance, desires, attachment, liking and needs.

When prana is moving upwards as we breathe, our brain is drawn to anything that we want. It "ignorantly" is drawn to the things that it believes will make us feel happy. A wise person recognizes that happiness is a source of inner peace and that lasting happiness can't be found in other objects or individuals.

In just in front of your spine, is the avadhuti Sushumna Shaking channel or singing channel. central channel. The name is a reference to the hum we experience when we experience true joy that rises up when prana flows freely across the Nadi.

The goal of "ha-tha" practice is to shift"ha "ha" along with the "tha" energies away from the side channels into the main channel. "Hatha" is originally used to push and pull the breath's inner energy to the center channel through manipulating the body's physical structure.

If prana flows effortlessly through this central channel, then we are at Samadhi and are considered to be in complete integration. It is marked by feelings of satisfaction pure joy and the wisdom.

These channels run around and connect at different central points across the body. These are called "wheels," and we refer to them as chakras. These charkas crossing the central channel and could transform into choke points, and stop prana movements. If you are hearing that someone is suffering from a blocked chakra, that means the central channel has been clogged by something inside some chakra.

The exact number and position of the chakras differs according to the different traditions. The majority of Hindu beliefs suggest there are the chakras are seven or six however, Buddhists believe there five.

Yoga and meditation can help unblock these points by shifting certain prana that is moving through the channels to the central channel. If you're doing yoga, you may feel an electric current that is moving across your body. When you feel the sensation of a "gut sensation" or "a feeling of a shiver" you're reacting to the sixth sense.

You can see the work prana is performing by looking at your breath. If prana's energy is moving via the correct channel it will be released through the right nostril. At this point the left, logical part of your brain is active. When you open your nose, it is the left. The right creative part of the brain becomes more dominant.

In most cases, there is one nostril that is stronger than the other. This can change every hour. If you've reached an absorption state either samadhi, nirvana or samad in meditation in meditation, you'll be able to breathe evenly through both nostrils at the same time. There is no energy moving through the channels to the sides.

One of the most effective methods to connect with the prana is to take note of specific sensations that you experience while breathing. It's not an accident that we connect our breath to joyful feelings, awake emotions, more energy and joy. When we exhale and exhale, we release sadness, sorrow and let go of the negative things that happen in our lives. The cycle of sadness and joy ever-changing and permanent is a circle that remains within us when we breathe.

If yoga pulls, pushes and moves the breath towards the central channel, by moving the body physically, meditation accomplishes exactly the same thing, by altering the mind. The ancient texts say that the thoughts of a person direct their prana just like someone is riding the back of a horse. This is why you can direct your prana by using your thoughts to move your thoughts towards that center point.

By practicing pranayama, meditation and pranayama, we can learn to control our breathing. Many people have noticed that meditation stops and breathing gets interrupted too. If we are in a state of rest and peaceful, we will not be able observe our breathing.

Since breath and thoughts are interconnected, they can be altered by focusing on only one. The yoga component involves controlling your breath performing exercises to control your prana using asanas and meditation. Pranayama practices that are properly executed can help treat illnesses and help us stay healthy. There are numerous techniques available that aid us in boosting our energylevels, relax and clear our minds, as well as to warm our bodies. A study from 2012 found that performing the ujjayi technique can shut off our stress response.

Through the combination of pranayama, meditation and asana with meditation and pranayama, your Kundalini energy, which is resting near the spine's base will start to flow upwards through the central channel. It will then flow by the chakra in the top of the head, which will bring your awakening. For some, this may take place only when they die. When our prana is sent to the heart chakra. It then releases through the crown chakra.

Because prana is an universal energy that doesn't exist in us, we're in no way separate from the fire's earth's, water's, or wind's energy around the world. The breath we breathe in our own body is connected to the breath outside.

As we become conscious of the prana that is in our bodies and breath as well as our body, we could also observe how energy flows throughout the world and impacts the weather and the environment as well as how intoxicants, caffeine, as well as food items we consume impact our energy.

Being conscious of prana and our body's subtle aspects can take us an entire life-time. When you meditate being aware of our thoughts can provide the appropriate circumstances to be able to act with wisdom. Becoming aware of blessings that prana offers us is the same skill. Through time and gaining more conscious awareness, we are able to deliberately shift our energy towards the central channel, and feel satisfaction and happiness that will never be interrupted.

There are many sources to help you maintain, sustain and improve the quality in your prana. They can be classified into four major categories: breath, calmness rest, food, and calmness.

You'll find higher levels of prana when you eat fresh food than you'll find in canned or stale food items. Foods that vegetarians consume are rich in prana however, because meat is dead it is regarded as negative or very low in prana.

The most potent prana source is breath. If you stop breathing and you die, you'll be dead. As I'll explain in a couple of minutes breathing patterns can have a profound impact on how we feel.

It was discovered that the quality and amount of prana as well as the way it moves through the channels of energy determines the state of mind we are in.

Since we don't pay sufficient focus on our channels of energy, they may be blocked, making the flow of prana to be sluggish or broken. This can lead to negative feelings, anxiety depression, anxiety, conflict anxiety, fear and worry.

In the event that our prana level is elevated and flow smoothly, in a steady and continuous manner Our minds will be positive and happy. and relaxed.

The ancient yoga texts provide definitions and descriptions of various techniques for pranayama.

In the Patanjali Yoga Sutra 2.49 defines pranayama as: in the following way: "In that state of being in asana or a posture that breaks the regular breathing or exhalation movements, pranayama is the regulation of breath."

This implies that prana is the life force that runs throughout the universe and that Ayama helps to extend or control it.

The ancient yogis realized how powerful breathing was and how it could boost the prana of a person. Therefore, they developed a unique breathing method which was able to boost the energy of a person, bring peace, promote well-being, and clear the minds to be more relaxed.

Pranayama isn't the best way in which you can control the way that your breathe is like some believe it is, however, it will help to control your prana, or energy through your breath. These techniques require breathing through your nose in an order where you breathe in and hold your breath and then exhale. The most popular breathing exercises are Nadi Shodhan, Bhramari pranayama and Bhastrika pranayama.

If done correctly the pranayama practice can help to bring harmony to your spirit body, mind, and spirit under supervision. This helps you to be mentally, spiritually, as well as physically robust.

The History of Pranayama

This timeline provides an overview of the history of pranayama and practices. While this list isn't designed to be exhaustive or complete It does contain textual sources that could be of interest to anyone who is interested in learning more about the history of pranayama.

"Brihadaranyaka Upanishad - 700 BCE"

Although prana's name was first discovered in the Chandogya Upanishad as early as 3000 CBE. However, the reference to a breathing technique is known as pranayama was not discovered until much later, about 700 BCE.

The first recorded mention of breathing through pranayama can be located in Brihadaranyaka Upanishad in the hymn 1.5.23. The breathing is a way of regulating the life force.

There are no other rules to practice pranayama that are not from the Upanishad. The idea that breathing can aid people attain immortality and improve their health is reiterated repeatedly in the yogic texts and teachings.

"The Bhagavad Gita - 5th Century to the 2nd Century BCE."

Pranayama is also included throughout the Bhagavad Gita. The chapter 4 text and verse 29 focuses on exhaling inhaling and exhaling conscious breath retention, and conscious exhaling to achieve a trancelike state. The text further states that regularly practicing pranayama will help someone gain greater control over their perception through "curtailing the process of eating."

"The Maitrayaniya Upanishad - Fourth Century BCE"

It's probably the most important pranayama book, since it has the first mention of pranayama in the context of a larger multifaceted system. It was likely written several hundred years prior to that of the Yoga Sutras of Patanjali, which taught the union of reasoning, meditation sensory withdrawal, concentration and breath control that is used in yoga.

Pranayama is explicitly mentioned in the chapter 6 in verse 21. It explains how you can achieve deliverance using various breathing techniques while the word "Om" to facilitate prana flow into your energy channels.

"Patanjali's Yoga Sutras - 100 to 400 CE"

Many scholars admit with the idea that this is an collection of the texts of all the early yoga teachers. At the time Patanjali became a yogi yoga had evolved and expanded to the extreme. While the Maitrayaniya upanishad mentioned the six-limbed system of yoga, it was expanded to include an eight-limbed system that included niyama asana Yama Pranayama, as well and four other stages of meditation that include Samadhi, dhyana, Dharana and pratyahara.

The text mentions pranayama in the verses 2.29 and 2.53 of the Sutras. Although Patanjali does not go into the depths of the meaning of prana, it describes specific aspects of breathing such as exhales, retention and the inhale. The book also discusses pranayama in the verse 2.51 which explains why it is different from all the other breathing techniques.

In addition, it outlines various benefits of pranayama. One of them is greater concentration and improved physical fitness. Concentration is the most heightened level of practice in yoga. In the verse 2.52 it explains the ways that pranayama practices can help to dissolve or reduce the veil that hides the "inner light."

The benefits of Pranayama

The secret to living an enjoyable and healthy life could be in the way you breathe. If you learn to pay attention to your breathing, it will help you return to the present, help you feel more relaxed and more aware of you.

Pranayama can cleanse the nadis, or psychic channels. It also helps to improve the physical and mental stability. It is capable of purifying more than 72,000 channels in the body. It is able to cleanse the blood and respiratory systems. Deep breathing is a great way to enrich your blood by supplying oxygen. Massive amounts of oxygen be delivered to capillaries, the heart, lungs and the brain.

Pranayama goes one step further than simply awareness of your breathing. It employs specific methods and rhythms to offer you a variety of benefits to your emotional, physical and mental state.

* Can slow down ageing process

* Revitalizes the body and mind.

* Immune system booster

* It is a source of positive energy and optimism.

* Energy boosts

It helps get rid of brain fog.

* Enhances attention and focus

* Helps reduce anxiety and worries.

* Calms the mind.

Pranayama practices can be helpful in treating many problems related to stress such as:

• Improving fitness through performing specific yoga asanas

* It can aid with losing weight

* Resets the cardiorespiratory systems and aids in lowering blood pressure.

* It assists in getting rid of any unnecessary thoughts and relax your mind and help to reduce anxiety and depression.

* It can help relieve asthma symptoms.

* Improve autonomic functions

Focusing your breath and paying attention to your breath can be extremely relaxing and rejuvenating.

Regularly doing this will improve your state of mind as well as memory and concentration

Psychology Today described breathing as "an extraordinary alternative to mindfulness you've haven't heard about." The magazine also noted that it "could assist those who cannot be passive since it's an active form of meditation."

There have been over 65 studies conducted on the combination of Sudarshan Kriya with pranayama breathing. They showed a myriad of health benefits.

Regulates Emotions

Pranayama breathing can assist a person to control their emotions. At a conference in Germany one of the founding members of the "Art of Living Foundation" Sri Sri Ravi Shankar, explained how breathing and emotions are linked.

If we are aware of the rhythm of our breathing, we are able to control our thoughts and manage negative emotions like jealousy, greed and anger, all while we're smiling from the heart.

* If you're part of the theatre You know that if the director requests you to increase your breathing speed it is possible to show you're in a state of anger. If you have to demonstrate your calm and peaceful mind, you'll be instructed to breathe slowly and slow.

* The breath is connected to emotions. There is a specific rhythm to your breathing for every emotion. While we're not able to control the emotion but you can manage these emotions by breathing.

A study conducted by Phillipot found that breathing patterns that resemble sadness, joy and anger, could cause the same emotion inside us.

This is the principle pranayama uses. Instead of letting emotions affect the way we breathe, we can alter our moods by learning to control our breathing. Because it's difficult to manage emotions, when we use pranayama techniques to control emotional states that are negative and overwhelming they can become an effective tool for enhancing our peace of mind and wellbeing.

Deep Breathing or Shallow Breathing

You can take a few minutes now and be aware of your breath. Are you feeling choppy, smooth or even shallow? Learn the correct breathing technique by watching the way newborn babies breathe. Have you noticed that their bellies move softly as their breaths come in and go out?

A majority of people breathe through their chests. This breathing style is shallow and sends the brain an indication that we're stressed and that something is not right. If we be taught to breathe deeply through our stomach, it will improve our breathing, ensuring the right amount of oxygen reaches the brain, and it tells it everything's okay.

You can take another few minutes to become conscious of your breathing for another time. While you've been contemplating it, has it become much more relaxed or longer?

The difference between breathing exercises and Pranayama

There are many people who call pranayama breathing exercises. However, not all breathing exercises is pranayama. The majority of breathe exercises do not qualify as pranayama. Pranayama refers to "expansion of the life force." it's purpose is to increase the body's capacity to store and increase prana within your body."

If we wish to improve the capacity to hold prana by pranayama, pranayama exercises will cleanse our nadis, which are energy pathways. Through regular practice of pranayama the channels become cleaner, and our bodies will be able to store more prana. In addition, our minds can be able to focus and focus more effectively. Pranayama practice regularly can help increase our spiritual power and bring joy, while also enhancing spiritual growth.

To enhance and preserve our vital force, pranayama uses five tools:

* Bandhas or locks

* External retention, also known as bahayia kumbhaka

Internal retention or antar Kumbhaka

* Exhalation Rehaka

Poorak or inhalation

When an exercise has locks or retentions are we able to discuss pranayama? The majority of breathing exercises that people practice are a simple form of pranayama. This can be achieved by eliminating the external locks and retention or by holding your breath after exhaling.

Regular breathing and Pranayama

Everyone is aware of breathing even babies. Today, the majority of us need to go to a breath class to cope with everyday life stress, anxiety and depression, driving and at work. Many people are aware that breathing deeply can be a way to ease stress and pressures, therefore we need to be aware of the practice of breathing pranayama.

Pranayama is a part of yoga that teaches us to regulate and extend our breathing in a variety of ways. It can help us learn to alter the rhythm of our breathing, the rate, and the depth in our breath.

Pranayama is being aware of your breathing. It is the correct deep, rhythmic, as well as slow breathing. It is a way to improve your respiratory system. It can calm your nervous system. It may help increase your concentration. The breath is a bridge between our mind, spirit and our body.

Your breathing rate can change in accordance with the conditions you. It could increase due to the emotional or physical stress and then slow down when you're relaxed and relaxed. If you are tired while taking a long walk then you'll feel breathless. Try this method to control your breathing so that you don't feel so tired. While climbing the stairs, make sure your shoulders are straight. Inhale slowly for two steps and then exhale for two steps. Keep a steady rhythm that is two breaths in, two breathes out. In this way you'll rid yourself of carbon dioxide, while getting more oxygen in, and you'll not get as exhausted.

In most cases you use only just a small portion of your lung's capacity when you breathe deeply. The ribcage doesn't expand completely. Your shoulders are typically in a slouche, and you're experiencing strain in the neck as well as your your upper back, due to the lack of enough oxygen in our bodies. This causes us to be tired and in a state of exhaustion. Make sure to keep your shoulders close without straining them and exhale in a slow and steady manner. Make sure that you force all oxygen out of your lung. Inhale and then stop. an easy, slow deep breath until your lungs are completely full. Take a deep breath by letting your nose out, but without lifting your shoulder blades. Keep doing this in as many instances as possible. While doing this your brain will be activated and will release tensions as you're giving your body more oxygen.

Different types of breathing

Abdominal Breathing: These is deep breathing in the abdominal area which brings sir to the biggest and lowest region of the lung. Breathing should be deep and slow to ensure that the diaphragm is utilized properly.

Thoracic Breathing , also known as Chest Breathing: You do this breathing by expanding and contracting by focusing on the chest and manage your abdomen. This fully activates the middle of the lungs.

Sectional Breathing or Clavicular Breathing Clavicular Breathing or Sectional Breathing: This is a low breathing technique in which your abdomen is controlled as you breath by pushing air to the upper portion of your lung. The shoulders and collar bones are raised , while your stomach is stretched when you breathe in.

A complete breath of pranayama will blend each of these. It starts by putting your stomach in the middle and then breathing through the thoracic region and onto the clavicular zone. The abdomen should expand as you breathe in and expand as you exhale. To understand this movement better, lie down in a meditative pose; Vajrasana would be best to place the hands of your stomach on. Breathe slowly and take a deep breath through the nose. Your hands should be separated from one another when your stomach begins to expand. Then, you'll keep your breath for a moment or two. Breathe slowly, until your stomach shrinks and pulls your hands closer. Take this breath for at least two seconds and repeat the breathing exercise five times. It's possible to do this in the form of breathing into your lungs for a period of four, holding for two seconds and then breathe out for eight counts and then hold for two seconds. Your breathing must be slow, rhythmic and deeply.

The lower part of your lungs will expand as you breathe. The diaphragm's rhythmic movements will gently massage your stomach, and help the organs perform better.

Pranayama is best practiced when sitting in a particular position like Ardhpadmasana as well as Padmasana and must be performed with a full stomach, and in the early mornings. Make sure you find an area that is well ventilated. Your breathing must be slow and rhythmic. Eyes must shut to manage your body and mind. You'll be using elements of poorka or inhalation and retention, also known as kumbhaka and exhalation, also known as rechaka.

Different kinds of Pranayama:

* Kapalabhati Pranayama This breathing method will allow air to escape your lungs somewhat forcefully however it will allow you to inhale slowly

* Bahya Pranayama For this breath, take a deep breath, exhale, and exhale, and then keep your breath

* Shitali Pranayama This is a cool breath

* Bhastrika Pranayama Breath: this breath draws air in and out.

* Brahamari Pranayama: This is the humming breath of bees.

* Anulom Vilom: This is a breathing technique that is used in alternate ways.

* Ujjayi Pranayama, this is the breath that has won

Breath and Mind

Your breathing patterns can reveal the state of your mind at present. It could be that you're feeling great about yourself and are planning to have a cocktail with a few acquaintances after work. Perhaps you're feeling overwhelmed due to trying to sort everything from the "inbox" to your "outbox" prior to the time your day's end.

Every stress can be good however if you operate constantly on high-octane you may be the perfect candidate for a major burnout. The short-term stress can be beneficial because it will assist you in completing that goal. If you are dependent on stress that is short-term every day, you could find that your body wears out. Your immune system is affected as well as your memory, focus and brain can be hampered by prolonged stress.

That's when your breathing takes over. It will restore your health. It will help you conserve energy for those times in your life that you'll need your mental strength.

Your breath can influence your brain and your mind. It is possible to learn a lot by learning to monitor your breathing and observe what's happening. Let's look at our nose. We have two nostrils. All we require is one big hole. There's a reason there are two nostrils. In the event that you blow your breath into your left nostril will stimulate your brain's right-side. In the event that you inhale through your left nostril, this engages the left side of the brain.

Researchers have discovered it is true that when breathing into the right nostril, the body's metabolism increases by more than twice the amount in the case of using the left nostril.

When the time we first came into this world, we breathed deeply before we began to cry. The last thing we'll do before our time is take a last breath, and after that, other people begin to cry. As you were born, it was you who shed tears while everyone else laughed. If you die you'll take your final breath, and the rest of us will be crying. If this doesn't happen it's because you didn't live the most fulfilling life.

Everyday we tend to forget about our breath. There are four energy sources:

* Calmness: This is a pleasant , happy state of mind

Breath: it is the most effective fuel source. Breathing can to energize our whole system. If you're feeling tired and need to relax, try deep breathing or alter the way you breathe and you may feel more energy.

* Try not sleep for more than a night to see how you feel the next day.

* Food: Fast for a couple of days, and you'll see that I'm talking about. If you consume too much or not enough it will deplete your energy

Simply taking a few minutes of meditation can boost your energy levels. Most people believe that meditation is the same thing as concentration, but that's not true. Meditation is the exact opposite of concentration. Concentration is what you will get when you meditate.

The Science Behind It

If you be observant and observe things carefully, you will see the rhythm of nature.

the seasons have an example of a natural rhythm. The body has also a rhythm. You might have noticed you feel hungry at exact times every day. You are tired simultaneously; this is called biorhythm. There is no one who is able to unlock your phone, except you.

It is possible to feel a rhythm to your breathing. It can be different in the day, in the night, and also when you feel different emotions. If you are feeling happy or are smelling the aroma of your favorite flower, then the breath will become intense steady, slow, and steady and your exhale will disappear. If you're unhappy or angry the exhale will be much more intense.

The rhythm of your thoughts is similar that runs through your thoughts patterns and your emotions. The way you breathe changes with the different emotions. It's different when you are feeling anger or anxiety. It is all dependent on how stressed you are as well as a pattern in the change that occurs within you.

Your breathing can create harmony with these rhythms. Eventually, the world becomes music. It takes about three days to master this. After you've learned it you'll only have to practice it for ten minutes a day. If you're in school and are preparing for an exam breathing exercises will help you to stay focused and increase your sensitivity.

Does stress impact longevity? Stress isn't the cause of death however it affects our health in a variety of ways. When stress hormones are elevated the risk of being prone to illness and disease. It is possible that you are living however, you're likely to get extremely sick. Relaxing your stress will help keep you healthy.

How can one use breathing and meditation techniques to manage anxiety or to reduce the negative effects of stress? There are many people who have found a way to manage their depression applying breathing methods. It is a good idea to use it as a substitute for taking antidepressants.

There has ever been a link between our thoughts as well as our breathing? This connection is as ancient like the relationship between breath and bodies. It dates all the way back to the very beginning of time.

The link has been present in every single ancient tradition. If you have the opportunity to observe the Maoris in New Zealand, they will greet each other by exchanging breaths. They will touch one another's nose, inhale and exhale. This is how they make connections and bring harmonious relationships between people.

Buddha advised us to pay attention to our breath, or Anapanasati. This will help you notice every feeling and allows you to reveal your true nature. The breath you breathe doesn't belong to an identity or religion. Every human being needs breath.

Breath and Life

Ancient yogis realized that breathing rate was correlated with the length of time we live as well as our overall health. They believed that in order to live until old age one must breathe in a slow and steady manner. To demonstrate this concept in greater specific detail, we're going to discuss our animal kingdom. Humans are classified as primates, such as apes and monkeys within the taxonomic classification. We can learn to breathe more efficiently through doing pranayama.

Never Pant Like Dogs

In the vertebrates, the tortoise that is the largest is likely to be among the oldest animals. The dogs breathe very quickly they are located on the opposite end on the scale. They live a short duration. Dogs breathe between 20 and 30 times per minute. They can live between 10 to 20 years.

The tortoise that is giant breathes 4 times per minute, and it can age 150 years. One of the oldest tortoises alive is believed to be around 250 years old. old. A tortoise called "Jonathan" is aged an age of 186 today and is the longest-living animal ever discovered. From now on when you notice you're breathing quickly and you are experiencing a tense breathing, take a few slow breaths.

Be Conscious, Breathe Slowly

We tend to take our breathing for granted since it's one of the many things can be done in a way that is automatic, such as the heart beating and our temperature remaining the same. All of this is determined by our nerve system and breathing isn't something that you need to be aware of each minute of the day. When used properly, it can aid in changing your life. Breath is a tool that can work on your mind and the body.

The ability to breathe more slowly can affect your mood positively. It reduces the amount of chemical reactions that occur when reacting to stress. It may boost the immune system within your body. When you are stressed, you'll usually be breathing shallowly through your chest. This could cause a lot of harm over time. If stress becomes chronic, then we must take action to avoid illness and discomfort. If you are able to control your breathing, then you have discovered the secret to your physical and mental well-being.

Even when you're exercising or simply running, it's best to keep your mind at ease as well as your tongue open. By focusing on breathing by your nostrils and out of your mouth , is the ideal method to tackle more difficult and more lengthy tasks.

If you breathe out and in by mouth, it taps the sympathetic nervous system, which triggers your fight or flight response. This is a good option if need to sprint and have to be as quick as you can, but breath breathing can reduce the body's ability to respond.

Slow breathing is healthy

The average human is breathing between 12-18 times per minute. This is the first thing that every first aid manual will teach you. Breathing for 12 seconds is okay, but once you get to 16 your body is feeling some strain.

With more advanced yoga practitioners and active, healthy people breathing normally, the rate of breath could be lower, leading to a longer life. A lower rate of breathing can lower stress on the heart and allow it to continue for a long time. When you incorporate exercises during breathing, it could make your body's capabilities harder to manage stress. The body's response to stress does have limitations. If it is time to stop, there's an event that shuts off hormones which aid in managing stress triggers. Your body will require some time to heal.

Pranayama Terminology

There are numerous terms that you've seen before and will be able to find through this text. To make sure that you know what they are, we'll review a few crucial words you should be aware of.

Ajapa The term Ajapa is a meditation method that focuses on the natural breath sound. It is an aspect of yoga. The word is derived in the form of "a," meaning "not," and "japa," which means "repeated." This means that the word translates to "not repeatedly repeated." In it's context, in this type of yoga japa means the laborious repeating of the sounds. This means that ajapa is an unrepeatable sound that is similar to the natural breath of a person. If you are able to regulate your breathing's sound using the practice of yoga. It is believed that it can generate feelings of kindness as well as peace, compassion and love.

Anasakti Yoga Anasakti Yoga Anasakti yoga can be described as a mode of life and a philosophy that was advocated by Mahatma Gandhi. It teaches people to not develop an obsession with the world of material things. Anasakti yoga will teach you how to release attachments that result from the actions of a person. According to the tradition, the absence of attachment can help people free themselves from suffering. The person who practices it won't be entangled by the attachments of the world of material things, helping them to live a life of eternal bliss. The person who practices this type of yoga remain committed and active in their activities and work however they do not have any desire to change the outcome.

Apana The word "apana" means "wind." Apana is the second most important Vayus, or prana types in Hatha yoga. Vayu in Sanskrit is "wind" and is a reference to the way that prana flows through your body. Apana vayu regulates prana's flow inwards and also controls the elimination of physical wastes as well as the elimination of toxins. It is located in the pelvic floor, and extends all the way to the lower abdomen, which regulates the reproductive function and digestion.

Arhatic Yoga Arhatic Yoga Arhatic yoga can be described as a technique that promotes spiritual growth designed to assist people in developing their lives faster, allowing them to be more effective in serving humanity as well as the Earth. The practice of yoga involves meditation, breathing asanas and spiritual practices which are brought together to form a cohesive system.

Ashtanga Ashtanga Ashtanga yoga, also known as yoga, is a physical yoga style that was developed by T. Krishnamacharya and Sri K. Pattabhi Jois. It is a derivative of Hatha yoga. Ashtanga is a reference to "eight legs" and is a reference to the eight-fold path , or eight yoga limbs that are described by the Yoga Sutras. It's a fluid flow that helps bring the body and the breath. This style emphasizes that you need to practice each daily.

Bhastrika Bhastrika Bhastrika refers to bellows breathing. It is a form of pranayama. It is considered to be among the most vital breathing methods. It's derived in the Sanskrit word meaning "bellows" due to the way the abdomen pumps air. It requires strong and rapid inhales as well as exhales that produce an audible noise. It helps cleanse the airways as well as increase the power of your mind and body.

Bindi Bindi Bindi is a symbol of protection, which numerous Hindus wear on the middle of their foreheads. The word comes from Bindu which is a reference to a dots or points. Bindu is the name given to the place that the creation process began and the bindi is a symbol of the beginning of creation. Traditionally, the bindi color is either red, white, or yellow.

Desa Desa Desa is Desa, a Sanskrit word which translates to country space, location, or place. In the traditional Indian tradition, desa is the same as the word "county. It is a unit of geo-cultural significance. In yoga, desa refers to the place in the body, especially in relation to breathing exercises. Desa can also be a method to treat any imbalance or disease that affect the body in Ayurveda.

Egoism is a term used to describe the behavior of a person who has egoism Egoism is a display of behavior driven by the self-interest of a person. It is also a reference to the notion that self-interest is the foundation of moral conduct.

Hasta Vinyasa - Hasta vinyasa is a sequence of actions in yoga that involve arm movements. It is derived from the words hasta, which means "formed by the hands" and vinyasa which means "coordinated motion."

Hatha Yoga - Hatha Yoga Pradipika was composed during the fifteenth century, by Swami Svatmarama. This is considered to be the oldest guidebook of Hatha yoga, and is considered one of three essential yoga manuals. Hatha yoga is designed to guide the practitioner through the body's awareness towards the Self's consciousness. It is comprised of asanasand pranayama as well as mudras, bandhas and Samadhi.

Kosha The Koshas are as the five layers of consciousness which conceal the real self. Each layer is revealed in bringing you closer to being one with the self and the world. Kash is a reference to "covering" also known as "sheath." This is why the koshas are commonly referred to as"the 5 sheaths.. The practice of yoga can lead an individual deeper into the self by utilizing the five koshas.

Kripalu Yoga Kripalu Yoga Kripalu Yoga can be described as a new yoga style that has been modified from the traditional Hatha practices. It consists of sequences of poses with no set order, and breathing and relaxation exercises. The aim of this yoga is to focus your attention inward and concentrate on the prana flow.

Kundalini is a term that means "coiled one." Kundalini refers to "coiled one." It's the primal force that is "coiled" in the bottom of your spine. Different yoga postures along with meditation, as well as guided breathing are able to you awaken the kundalini and help open your chakras.

Manipura Manipura Manipura is the title given to the chakra in the solar plexus. Mani means "gem," while Pura is a reference to "city." The literal translate the word to "city filled with jewels." This allows us to see the chakra as our personal treasure, and the center of our health.

Mudra Murda Murda is a sacred and symbolic gesture, which is used in yoga. A very famous mudras can be used in yoga and meditation to aid in the channeling of prana. It is a signifying the act of sealing, gesture, or mark. In various religions and traditions there are approximately 400 mudras. Each one is unique in symbolism and considered to be able to create a particular influence on the mind as well as the body.

Nadi Nadi Nadi is a Greek word meaning flow or tube or channel. It is the system of channels that your energy flows through. The number of nadis one has is contingent on the culture, but there are three main nadis which move through the spinal cord as well as chakras.

Pavan The word "Pavan" Pavana is a word that means air, which is the fifth element in the universe. According to the Hindu belief, the five elements will disappear after death. Other elements include Aakash (sky), Agni (fire), Jala (water) and Bhumi (earth).

Pingala The Pingala Pingala is one of the nasal nadis in the Astral Body. It's located in the right nostril, and extends through the chakra of root. It is located on one side of the spine. It is rational, objective and analytical. It can also be aggressive.

Prana Prana Prana is Prana is a Sanskrit word that has many English translations, such as vitality, vital energy as well as life force. It is a reference to all the energy manifesting that exists in the universe. It is found in living creatures as well as inanimate objects.

Rasa - Rasa means fluid, sap, or essence. Spiritually, it is the core of human experience. It's the emotion which govern our lives. Tantric beliefs contain nine fundamental human emotions. In yoga there are only three rasas. rasas are considered to be essential.

Samadhi is the last step on the yoga path. It is a reference to freedom, bliss and awakening. It is a key concept in Buddhism and Hinduism it is considered as the ultimate goal of all spiritual and intellectual activities.

Shodhana Shodhana - This Sanskrit word is a synonym for cleaning or purifying. It is usually paired with Nadi. Nadi Shodhana is a relaxing breathing exercise that helps reduce stress, tension, and fatigue.

Sitali - Sitali - Sanskrit word means cool or soothe. It is typically used to describe a type of pranayama. Sitali is when tongues are stretched out, and breath is drawn in through the tongue, as if it were straws.

Tantra Yoga Tantra Yoga Tantra is a kind of yoga that utilizes different practices to discover the universe by looking at it from the human microcosm. It is a way to balance our instincts and help us reach enlightenment.

Tapasya Tapasya Tapasya literally means "generation of energy and heat." It requires self-control and moderation, as well as deep meditation, and the effort to attain self-realization. The monks and gurus of Hinduism, Jainism, and Buddhism follow this path to achieve spiritual freedom.

Yogini is female yoga masters. The male version is Yogi. It is a reference to the goddess of light.

Yuj Yuj Yuj is a word that means join. The word yoga is from, and is a physical, mental and mental discipline that was developed in the ancient world of India. Yuj is yoga's word of origin which means yoga's goal is to connect the body, spirit and mind.

Precautions

There are a few precautions you must take prior to beginning pranayama.

* Do not practice pranayama when your lungs are clogged.

* Be sure to do pranayama in a space which is air-conditioned or do it outside.

* Never do pranayama in a hurry.

* If you are a regular practitioner of asanas and pranayama, you should do your asanas prior to doing pranayama. When you've completed your asanas then relax into the Shavasana posture prior to doing your pranayama. Do not exercise after you've completed your pranayama.

* Never practice pranayama if you feel tired. Take a break for 15 minutes in Shavasana posture prior to doing the pranayama.

* If you feel fatigue or discomfort you should stop pranayama. Lay down in Shavasana with your breathing normal. Speak to a yoga instructor before you begin the pranayama.

* If you're new to pranayama it is best not to be able to hold your breath. Once you're confident with pranayama's basics it is possible to breathe under the guidance of an expert who has mastered the basics of yoga breathing.

* It will help if you didn't practice pranayama immediately after having had a meal. It is recommended to wait for around three hours after eating. Large meals will take longer to digest. If you practice pranayama at night take a nutritious snack that is digestible prior to the time you start your pranayama.

Do not make sounding noises while breathing. Keep your breathing constant and steady.

* Never do pranayama exercises that cause strain. The lungs are extremely delicate. Be sure that your breathing doesn't exceed the limits of your lungs.

Make sure to breathe in through the nose, unless you are instructed not to.

* Pranayama should be done once you've gained control of your body through mastering all of the poses. Pranayama practice will create the body with energy as yoga poses help to eliminate any blockages that stop the body's energy moving.

* If you have chronic medical condition, consult your yoga instructor or doctor prior to starting pranayama.

If you suffer from hernia or high blood pressure or heart condition and you are not able to perform bhastrika and Kapal Bhati pranayama. If you're doing the kapalabhati method and are just beginning practice, ensure you exhale slowly and avoid using excessive force.

If you suffer from an abnormally low blood-pressure, do not do pranayama skitkari. Don't do this pranayama during the winter months.

Don't do suryabhedi during the summer season.

Do not do chandrabhedi in those wintery months.

* Individuals with an abdominal hernia or have high blood pressure shouldn't do the

agnisar pranayama. Do not practice this pranayama if having surgery for the stomach.

Chapter 12: Importance Of Proper Breath

I wrote in the introduction that we humans aren't breathing correctly. If we're not physically exhausted the majority of us do not think about our breathing. This is why a lot of us breathe incorrectly and only use about 1/3 of our lung capacity. Researchers have discovered that this may be the root of many health problems. If we aren't breathing fully we feel tired stressed, anxious, depressed overwhelmed and it affects our sleep.

In just a day, we breath around 20000 times. It aids the cardiovascular, immune and digestive, muscular and nerve systems. About 70% of the contaminants in our body are eliminated via our breathing. The main function of the lungs is to transport oxygen in our air into get into the red blood cells in our bodies. Red blood cells transfer oxygen around the entire body. The lungs also aid in eliminate CO_2 after exhaling.

There are many breathing mistakes that cause people to constrict their lung capacity. They include:

* Consciously breathing, you are holding your breath.

The signs that you are holding your breath could include sighing more frequently than usual and is the body's way to get more oxygen, particularly when you're stressed or anxious. tension. It is likely that you will take taking a deep breath, and you will you will feel tension in your shoulders and neck.

• Breathing with your mouth

Breathing through your mouth instead of through the nose is a common practice that can make you be tired and cause dry mouth. If you're not breathing well by using your nostrils, you may change your blood pressure as well as heart rate. Additionally, it increases the stress response. It is made in the nasal passages, which when inhaled, dramatically enhances the capacity of their body to take in oxygen. This is vital during exercise.

To help you determine whether you're breathing correctly or not, here are the four signs that indicate improper breathing. Then, you'll discover six tests that you can take to determine if you are breathing in a way that is not correct.

The first indication of poor breathing is typically crying. The reason for yawning is typically when you're tired but it can also be triggered by a shortness of breath or breathing shallowly. This is particularly true in cases of obesity or have health issues.

Another sign is when you grind your teeth when you're asleep. If you breath in a way that is not correct, it's often coupled with teeth grinding as both are typical signs of stress.

The third indicator is that you are experiencing tension in your neck and shoulders. About 80% of us breathe through the upper chest. When we don't take deep breathes we take short breaths that cause the muscles in the shoulders, back, and neck to compensate, and then tighten to allow the body to breathe deeper , so that the lungs be able to take in more oxygen.

The fourth indication is that you are always exhausted. The most commonly observed consequence of improper breathing is that you are exhausted because you aren't able to access the right amount of your respiratory system.

With that in mind we'll try these tests to identify incorrect breathing.

1. Breathing in the upper chest

You'll lie on your back, and put one hand on your chest. The other hand will be placed on the top of your body while the other is on your stomach for this test. You will lie here for a couple of minutes and observe the way the hands of your body move. If your chest's hand can be moved when you breathe however, the hand on your belly does not move, then you're an air-breather. Any more than a small movement of your chest suggests that you're not breathing properly.

2. Breathing in shallow breath

You will lay on your back to perform this test. Place your hands on your lower ribs, with one hand placed on either side. While breathing in, you should feel a smooth expansion of the ribs when you breathe in , and then a slow recoil when you exhale. If your ribs do not move the way you expect, then your breathing is far too slow, even though you feel the belly expanding.

3. Breathing in excess

When you're still lying on your back Take a few moments to let your body get into a comfortable breathing rhythm. Start to measure how long your next exhale , and then measure the length of the next breath is. Your exhale should be a little longer. If it's not, you're an over drinker. To test for a second time you can try to cut down on the length of your inhale. If you experience any kind of discomfort, you're probably an over-breather. Since it's easy to alter how these tests go it is possible to have someone else perform the test for you in a moment when you're not paying attention.

4. Breath Inhalation and Holding

Holding your breath when you breathe in is likely to be one of the most common bad breathing patterns. To find out the reason pay attention to the time between exhale and inhale. The breath-holder is likely to experience an "catch" and could be able to see that they struggle to begin the exhale. This can be especially apparent when you are exercising. It can be reduced by conscious relaxation of the stomach at the time that the inhale is over.

5. Breathing Reverse

A reverse breath occurs when the diaphragm is pulled towards the chest during inhalation and falls out as you exhale. Place your body on the floor and put an arm on your stomach. The belly should gradually fall flat when you breathe out, and rise when breathe in. If it's the reverse it means you're reverse breathers. Since this kind of breathing is more likely to occur when you're exerting yourself however, it's not 100% reliable.

6. Mouth Breathing

It's pretty simple to recognize if you're an oral breather. If you're not certain the only thing you have to do is talk to your friend to help you or look at yourself while you're not focusing on your breath.

Those exercises serve a purpose. You need to be aware of the way you breathe. That means you are able to actively improve the issue. This is important as breathing has a larger effect on the health of our body than many realize. Breathing is so vital that the human race has long noted the value of breathing for survival, and how our mind and body function.

In the early millennium BCE the two faiths Tao and Hinduism place a high value on the concept of a "vital concept" that circulates across us as a kind of energy. They also saw breathing as its manifestation. In Tao the concept of this principle is called Qi. In the Hindus call it prana according to what we've discovered.

A little later it was discovered that later, the Greek phrase pneuma and the word ruah Hebrew was a reference to God's breath and presence. In Latin related languages, spiritus is the basis of breathing and spirit. Pranayama was the first type of breath retention based upon the concept of managing the respiratory system to improve longevity.

Johannes Heinrich Schultz, a German psychiatrist, invented "autogenic therapy" during the 20th century in order to help people to relax. The method was based on breathing slowly and deeply and is most likely to be one of the most popular breathing methods. Many modern types of mindfulness meditation focus on breathing exercises.

Every relaxation, meditation or calming method is based on breathing, which might be the most common factor in all methods to soothe the body and mind. The study of physiology and effects of breathing control gives proof of the benefits of controlling and monitoring our breathing. Even if only an understanding of the basics of physiology, it will help you understand how controlled breathing can cause relaxation. We all know that our emotions influence our bodies. When we're feeling content our corners of the mouth will rise while the corners of our eyes will curl to create a distinctive expression.

The autonomic nervous systems, or ANS connects the brain with the body via a two-way street. If you're feeling nervous or stress over things that are happening in your life, your brain is able to activate your sympathetic nervous system by its nerves in the ANS. This is is known as the"fight or flight" response. It causes your heart rate to increase and your breathing to get more intense and, in addition, increase your breathing.

Similar to that, when you're secure and peaceful and relaxed or doing things that are enjoyable your breath will become more pronounced and then slow. This happens because you are being influenced by your parasympathetic nervous system that creates a calming effect. The thing that isn't as well known is that the effects occur in opposite directions. The health of your body can influence the way you feel. Researchers have discovered that when you smile the brain responds in the same way. That means that you'll begin to feel more positive emotions. Breathing can have the same kind of impact.

The lungs and heart send our brains signals and let them know that everything is fine even when they're not. The way in which this happens is through the connection between the heart and lungs and the nerves they carry. Each time the air you breath in your heart is instructed to beat a little faster. Inhaling the heart, it slows down by a little. In the end, you will notice a small shift in your heart rate each minute.

If you choose to decide to make one phase of the cycle longer than the other and continue to do this for a short period of time and the cumulative effects will either increase or lower the heart rate. If you let your inhale last for a short time the heart rate will rise. This is due to it sending an alert to the brain that you are more active in your brain and body, activating your sympathetic nerve system. This is not the case when you make your exhales more prolonged. The parasympathetic nervous systems gets activated, and the body informs the brain that everything is healthy and will slow up the entire body.

It is noticeable in people with breathing issues. When the problems are acute or intermittent, they can result in a panic attack. If they're chronic and persistent, they can trigger mild anxiety. The research suggests that approximately 60% of those suffering from COPD have depression issues or anxieties. These conditions are most likely rooted in worries about what the disease could do to them, but mechanical causes can also be a factor in this. The discomfort they feel frequently leads to faster breathing, which isn't compatible the oxygen supply that they need but can increase their physical and mental discomfort and anxiety.

Rapid breathing can be a catalyst to trigger and contribute to anxiety attacks by fears that trigger, which triggers rapid breathing that can increase anxiety. Georg Alpers, in 2005 and with the assistance by his associates, witnessed an increase in unconscious hyperventilation as someone who was averse to driving went out on the road.

The anxiety is due to breathing issues or any other issue the anxiety can be reduced by using a variety of breathing techniques that are derived from Eastern methods. For instance, focusing on your breath is a method which focuses your attention on the breath, and is among the initial elements that mindfulness meditation. When you mix reassuring thoughts with breathing you will be able to control your nerve system.

The findings of research suggest that the vagus nerve as well as certain neurotransmitters in the brain are the factors behind the effects changes in breathing can have on heart rate. Keep in mind it is that your ANS is trying to ensure that your background systems are well-balanced and functioning correctly to the constantly changing conditions of the day.

Nadi and Svara

Svara can be described as a breath method that assists you in controlling your breath by changing breathing patterns through the left and right nostrils. The purpose of this technique is to regulate the flow of prana throughout your channels of energy, the nadis to help you attain physical, spiritual, and mental wellness.

Svara is Sanskrit which means sound or tone. There are two major nasals. The Ida and Pingala and represent the flow of air through the left and right nostrils. Yogis have discovered that by this physical connection between the ida and Pingala it is possible to influence the mental and vital energies within your body to activate sushumna. This is how they devised different methods to balance the svara. There are a variety of methods that can help balance the svara but the primary one is the nadi shodhana pranayama. It is meant to cleanse the fine energy network of the nadi within the body. This is also called alternate nostril breathing.

By pranayam you create an breathing pattern that flows through your left and right nostrils and concentrate on the way air is moving through your nose. There are several stages of this, from basic to advanced however the basic principle remains that this breathing pattern balance cleanses and energizes the energy of the body and mind. There are other more specific pranayamas like the surya bheda in which the Pingala is stimulated when you breathe through your right nostril. Chandra Bheda occurs where the ida is stimulated by breath through your nose alone.

Diaphragmatic Breathing

Diaphragmatic breathing is an individualized breathing method that requires you to breathe deep breaths that fully engage the diaphragm. The diaphragm muscle is a dome situated beneath the lungs. It is responsible for controlling your respiratory function. When you breathe in the diaphragm, it's pushed down. This simple motion will result in the basis of a sequence of happenings. Your lungs will begin to expand, which creates negative pressure, pulling air into your nose and mouth. As you begin to let go of the breath, your diaphragm begins to raise and help eliminate all air out of your lungs.

Poor posture, stress tight clothing, stress, and other conditions that weaken your breathing muscles can lead people to develop into breathing through their chests. There is evidence diaphragmatic breathing may aid people suffering from COPD. Diaphragmatic breathing is when you're fully engaging your diaphragm, stomach, and abdominal muscles while you breathe.

If you're here, then you'll probably want to know how to do diaphragmatic breathing. This easy technique will give you a solid foundation for what you can expect from breathing techniques of pranayama.

Relax into a comfortable sitting positionor lay down. If you opt to join a chair sure that you've got your feet level with the floor, and ensure that your shoulders, head and neck are in a relaxed position. It is not a good idea to let your back straight until you feel uncomfortable. Likewise, you shouldn't also be sitting in a slump. If you're lying down, put an extra pillow between your knees and head to make you more comfortable. You can bend your knees as you want to.

Put the hands of one on your chest. While you breathe and correctly using your diaphragm muscles your hand should be in a steady position while you breathe. Put your other hand underneath your ribcage. The epigastric area that you feel will assist you to feel your diaphragm while you breathe.

Inhale slowly by rubbing your nose. You want the air coming via your nostrils to move to the lungs, to cause the belly to rise. Be sure not to over-stress or push your abdominal muscles out. The flow of air and the movement to be easy. It should only be used in the epigastric region. You shouldn't feel like you're forced to push the low-abdomen to go out by pushing the muscles. Also, you shouldn't feel your hands on your chest move as much.

Breathe by mouth. Allow your stomach to ease into itself. Your belly should slide inwards. Do not force your stomach to come in by clenching or pulling your muscles. Be sure to exhale slowly and with slightly closed lips. Also, the hand that rests on your chest should be nearly still.

If you notice it difficult to breathe initially, it's probably due to your habit of to breathing using your chest. Although the frequency with which you perform this exercise will depend on the health of your body, it's generally performed three times in the beginning. A majority of people opt to practice it for 5 to 10 minutes and up to four times a throughout the day. If at any time you begin to feel dizzy or lightheaded, end the breathing practice and lie down, if you're not already. This is thought as a natural method to breathe.

As diaphragmatic breathing assists you to connect the diaphragm and bring you many advantages, such as:

* Encourage relaxation

* Reduce oxygen demand

* Lower heart rate and blood pressure.

* Improve core muscle stability

* Strengthen the diaphragm.

The diaphragmatic breathing technique has been acknowledged to be beneficial to people suffering from asthma and COPD however, it shouldn't be used as a sole treatment. It may also aid in reducing anxiety, however if it is done wrong, it could aggravate the symptoms. Patients with respiratory issues need to be cautious when they begin to practice this kind of breathing. It could start with more fatigue and even a sluggish breathing. It is recommended that you started slowly to reap the advantages.

Breathing Postures

When you begin the next chapter's pranayama methods You will need to be aware of the position you'll be using. There are a variety of yoga poses that you can choose from. Here we will go over some of the popular postures you can do for pranayama.

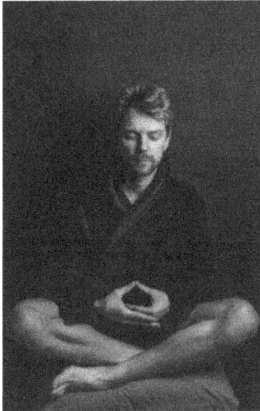

Simple Pose (sukhasana)

The easiest pose is the ideal posture for beginners or for anyone who's not practiced yoga before. The name "easy pose" is because of a reason. Simple pose is a standing position with a cross-legged back. It's the one that most students in grade school sit in when they are in circle.

Place your feet on the floor or on your mat with your legs spread out towards the front while keeping your body straight in order to achieve this position. The right foot slowly folds underneath your left leg, and then put the left foot underneath your right thigh. The legs should meet at mid-shins instead of at the ankles. Move your buttocks to ensure that you're on your sit bones and ensure your spine is aligned. You may also put an bolster or pillow under your buttocks in order to lift your hips in case you are feeling any discomfort.

It is an ideal pose for anyone however, if you suffer from knee issues, like knee surgeries or arthritis it might not be the ideal. Additionally, if you suffer from an injury to your back, you might not be able in this position for more that five minutes.

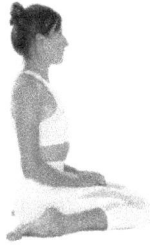

Hero Pose (virasana)

This is a bit more complicated than a simple pose, so it's might not be the most suitable option for people who are new to yoga.

In order to get into this posture begin by kneeling down in the ground. You can put the bolster or a an unrolled blanket in between your calves and thighs should you require. Make sure your thighs remain perpendicular to your floor and connect your inner knees. Move your feet forward in a way that they are slightly larger that your hips. Your feet's tops should rest on the floor.

Inhale, then slowly return to the middle. Your torso should lean towards the forward. Put your thumbs in the knee bend and then pull the muscles of your calf toward your heels. After that, you can sit between between your feet.

If you notice that your buttocks do not rest comfortably on the floor lift them up on a sturdy block or book that is put between your toes. The bones in your sitting position must be supported evenly. There should be a thumb's width space between your heel and your outer hips. In turn, bring your thighs forward and press the top part of the bones in your thigh to the floor. Your hands should be on your lap.

Lift your sternum up and take your shoulders and roll them up and down your back. Then, extend your tailbone towards the floor until you're securely anchored into your body.

This pose should be performed with caution for those who suffer from heart issues or headaches. It is also recommended in the event of knee or ankle injuries. If you have injuries then, you should stay clear of this posture unless you receive some help by a teacher.

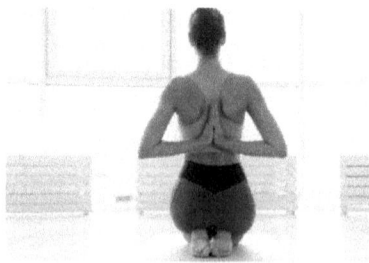

Thunderbolt Pose (Vajrayana)

This is a traditional and traditional seated posture that is like the hero pose we've done earlier. It is possible to move into this posture the same way as in the hero pose however, the only thing you should not do is split your feet. Your heels must remain in contact and your buttocks should rest on top of them.

Begin by kneeling down with your hips and buttocks elevated off your legs. If you're in need of additional padding, you can place blankets under your shins, feet, and knees. Your thighs must be straight to the floor and your inner knees must be in alignment.

Take your toes out of the sock as you keep your toes in the floor. After exhaling, you can come to your feet and rest. Your shins and feet should be aligned and your feet should not be splayed open or tucked into.

Maintain your back straight, and lift your shoulders and then back down to ease into the position. Keep your collarbones open and stretch your tailbone toward the floor.

Similar to the hero pose, it is best avoided in the event of an ankle knee or ankle injury.

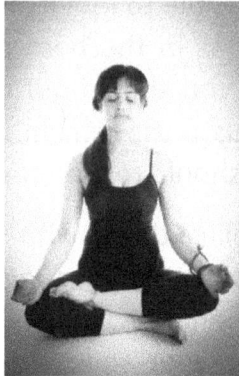

Half Lotus Pose (Ardha padmasana)

Everyone thinks of the lotus pose when it comes to sitting yoga, however it's more complex and poses that not everyone can do. It is a good idea to try the half lotus posture. While it's less difficult than the lotus posture however, it is too challenging for complete beginners.

In order to get yourself into this posture begin by sitting on the floor, with your legs straight towards the front and you spine straight.

Relax your right knee and wrap it around your chest. Then , bring your right ankle to the hip crease on your left in a way that your bottom foot is pointed toward the sky. The top of your foot should rest against the hip crease.

Let the left knee bend and then lower the left leg underneath the right knee.

Check that your spine is straight and that your shoulders are in a relaxed position.

This pose is not recommended in case you've had recent ankle, hip and knee injury. If your knees, ankles or hips are stretched, you might be unable to cross your legs. Do not push yourself into this position.

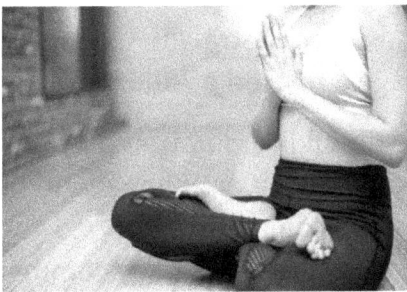

Lotus Pose (padmasana)

To begin this posture to begin, sit on the floor, with your legs spread in front of you with your spine straight.

Then bend your right knee, and then externally rotate your hip until your knee falls towards the left. Bring your right leg into your left hand, and then place the knee into your left hand. Your foot should rest on the line on your leg's left side. Press the foot's top into the crease of your hip. The right knee should sit on your floor.

Begin by leaning back. Then, you will begin to bend your left knee and then draw your left foot toward your right knee. Keep the left ankle by your hand, and slowly move your left heel towards the hip crease on your right side.

Keep your back straight and keep your shoulders in a relaxed position.

This pose shouldn't be attempted by anyone who is new to yoga or anyone who has knee, ankle, or hip pain. Do not try to force your legs into this posture. It is recommended to walk slowly and with care and stop when you feel any kind of discomfort.

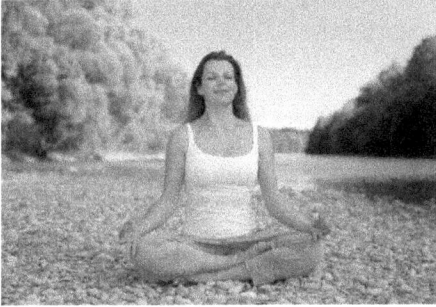

Exciting Pose (swastikasana)

This is an easy post to learn and is able to be held for longer periods. Some find it more difficult than a simple poses.

In order to get in this position, begin by sitting on the ground with your legs extended to the sides. Begin in folding your right leg over and then place the sole of the left leg against the inner thigh of the other leg.

Relax your right leg and put your right foot in the space between your muscles of the left thigh and calf. Keep your left foot in place by the toes, then slowly lift it and place it between your right thigh and the calf.

Make sure your knees are on the floor.

This pose should not be attempted for those with sacral infections or have issues with sciatica, which can squeeze the nerve.

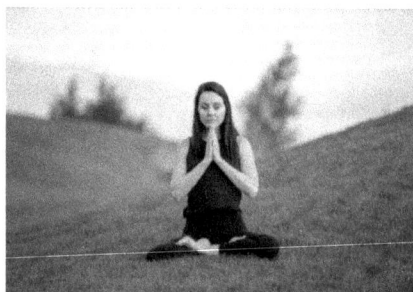

Achieved Pose (siddhasana)

It is a simple yoga pose that is suitable for beginners. To begin the practice begin by sitting on the floor and crossing your legs. Set one foot near the inner thigh. Then bring the other foot to the ankle until both heels are almost at the midline.

Be sure you have your spine straight, and that your shoulders at a comfortable level. If you're unable to do this put a blanket on your knees, hips or your hips.

As with the easy and auspicious posture Be cautious if you suffer from sciatica, knee or hip issues.

Selecting the Best Pose for You

You should choose the ideal pose for yourself and your body to accomplish. Do not attempt to force yourself into a posture and you are only likely to create more issues. If any of the poses we've discussed do not suit you then you are able to be in a chair making sure that your back is not pressed against any part of your chair's back.

If you're healthy in your ankles and hips, you could attempt any of the postures. The most frequently used pose is the easy one. It is essential you keep in mind that for a long-lasting energy-boosting, healthy and healthy experience, you must choose an appropriate position that allows you to feel at ease.

Chapter 13: Pranayama Breath

Before you start your pranayama breathing routine it is important to understand the fundamental guidelines for the practice. Let's review the basics of these guidelines to ensure that you're prepared.

1. It's not a bad idea to try some stretching exercises to warm your body and get your breathing flowing.

2. Make sure to breathe through the nose , unless instructed not to or if you are suffering from an obstruction to breathing. When you breathe in, your abdomen should contract when you inhale. The chest should move only little by breathing.

3. Be sure your nose, face, and mouth are all relaxed.

4. Don't force your breath , or retention to last longer than is normal. If you attempt at imposing it it's only going to agitate your mind.

5. It is best if both nostrils are open to the same degree. If one side appears as if it's closing, you can try lying to the side on your back for 30-60 minutes.

6. Be sure to know your limitations. You can overdo simple pranayama. It's possible it's not the appropriate method for you. If you feel

out of place or irritable, you may be nervous, or agitated you should stop and go back to the normal breathing.

With this in mind what is a complete yoga breath cycle? Let's discover. Yoga breaths that are full of yogic energy begin with fluid and deep breaths that cover three different areas of your torso separately. In the beginning, you fill the abdomen's lower part. Then, the mid-section the torso is filled with breath, thereby expanding the diaphragm and the ribs. Finally, the breath will fill up the shoulders and chest just when the inhale is coming close to an end. The purposeful and slow inhale is followed by a lengthy, slow exhale that releases the breath from the three parts and in reverse. The entire yoga breathing will consist of one full inhale, and a complete exhale.

You must ensure that both your inhale as well as exhale are both fluid and continuous. You should never ever feel any tension. Be aware that it may take some time to establish an easy practice of pranayama. This is especially when you've never tried pranayama before. That's why pranayama is often regarded as a practice. The most important thing is setting the intention of building the ability to breathe deliberately effortlessly, without tension or struggle.

To fully practice yogic breathing practice full yogic breath, follow these steps:

1. Find a comfortable position to sit in. Be sure the pelvic bone is securely anchored in the floor below the weight of your body and you have a straight spine. It is also possible to lie on your back if you like.

2. Shut your eyes, and allow time to relax. Close your mouth and breathe through your nose. Relax your mind and concentrate on breathing naturally. Be present in the moment.

3. Once you're ready, take a deep breath slowly and with a purpose. Begin to draw the breath deeply into the abdomen's lower part, beginning at the pelvic floor and let it slowly expand to the navel, then out, out away from your spine. Concentrate first on filling your lower abdomen.

4. While filling this area by breathing Let it expand to every direction in the direction of the navel.

5. When this area is fully filled, inhale to fill your mid-torso. Keep drawing the breath upwards from the navel upwards to the ribs, then let the breath expand the diaphragm, ribs and the mid-back.

6. After you've filled your mid-torso area with breath, finish your exhale through drawing your breath up into the chest area above to fill the sternum and the heart, then your shoulders as well as the back on the neck. The collarbones will rise a little.

7. Relax and allow the natural pause which occurs at the top of your breath to occur. You can then let go of the slow and long exhale. Let the breath go from the chest's upper region and to the mid-torso and then emptying the abdomen of the lower part. The belly will relax and draw into.

8. Your exhale can be followed by an unnatural pausing. This should happen prior to starting your next cycle.

Try this for several times for up to 15 minutes. After that, let your breath be restored to normal, before you open your eyes.

Making preparations

Before you begin any pranayama exercise you must prepare yourself. The first thing be aware of is when in the the day that you are planning to do the pranayama. Pranayama is typically practiced before dawn. It is at this time of the morning where the body is relaxed while the mind remains relaxed. To get up earlier than usual would like will mean going to sleep earlier. It is also important to remove distractions like TV and other gadgets to encourage relaxation. Do not fret, however in the event that mornings are ideal for you, cool practices like ujjayi Nadi dirgha, and shodhana can be performed before bed.

Consistency is more important than the time. Be sure to choose the most appropriate time to practice. Even if you are able to take ten or fifteen minutes however long as you're able to perform it every day, that's what matters. It is recommended to perform your pranayama in the same time each day. It is best to do it at the same time helps you develop the discipline needed to keep practicing it.

If you're in a place the pranayama practice should be done in a space that is ventilated. Be sure to not practice under the shade of a fan or near an air conditioner as it can distract you and cause the chills. Try to keep your space clear. This space should be sacred to yourclean and secure. If you are able practice outside, do so in the event that the weather is suitable and you aren't suffering from allergies that can hinder the practice.

Make sure you don't eat anything for at least three or four hours prior to the time you practice. This is why you should practice early at the beginning of your day is ideal. It's difficult to practice breathing exercises when you are on a an over-full stomach. What you eat as well as the quantity of food you consumed and the time you had dinner the night before will impact your pranayama practice the next day.

You must ensure you've got rid of any distracting devices. You must turn off your phone, not just turn them on to vibrate, then remove them. It is also necessary to switch off and store away tablets and computers to avoid being interrupted. If you have family members or neighbors who drop-in or call them regularly, inform them about what you're doing and tell them not to interrupt your work.

If you're menstruating the practices of nadi-shodhana or dirgha and ujjayi can ease cramps and other symptoms as well as decreasing fatigue. If you're pregnant consult your physician and consider joining the prenatal yoga class.

Before you exercise, you should do a nasal cleanse. Neti Pots are likely to be the most efficient method to accomplish this.

It's not difficult to keep up with your routine. These guidelines show you how to begin and what might lead you to quit practicing. Use the guidelines to help ensure that you're well-prepared to prevent any potential mistakes before they occur.

Purification of Nadis

In the human body, 72,000 Nadis carry prana through various parts of the body. However, impurities may cause Nadis to cease working. The first step is to activate the Nadi before it is possible to purify them so that they can allow prana to flow once more.

Pingala and Ida Nadis are activated by breath-based techniques, such as pranayama. If you deliberately breath in or out using only your right nostril it activates it to activate the

Pingala Nadi. If your breath in or out using only your left nostril it triggers the Ida Nadi.

To awaken Sushmna you must reach a balance between the two Nadis. When you have reached the right balance between these Nadis, it could assist in the process of an Kundalini awakening. If you fail to attain a equilibrium, Sushumna will remain closed and Kundalini will be inactive. Pingala the equilibrium of Ida are achievable only after tiny nadis, also called Nadikas connected to these two Nadis, are cleansed somehow.

It is essential to take part in Nadi Shuddhi Pranayama prior to yoga in order to cleanse your nadis. If impurities impede the Nadis, prana shakti is unable to traverse your Nadis. Nadi purification is done by two methods:

1. Smanu is a mental procedure that requires you to repeat the Bija mantra

2. Nirmanu This is the physical cleansing of Shatkarmas as Dhauti Kriya.

Samanu is a more advanced form of yoga which will help flush out impurities. The samanu routine is typically performed while sitting in lotus position however if you are unable to effortlessly do that pose pick one of the others we talked over in the past. When you do this, you'll be repeating Vayu Bija Mantra repeatedly. This mantra is "yam." It is a more advanced method therefore, it might never be something that you would want to try if you're brand new to yoga, pranayam or other similar methods, so proceed with care.

1. Keep the right nostril in close Breathe through the left nostril, while mentally repeating "yam" 16 times.

2. Take a deep breath each moment and then mentally repeat "yam" for another 64 times.

3. Close your left nostril and breathe in through your right nostril while repeating "yam" 32 times.

After that, you'll using then the Agni Bija Mantra. This will use the Agni Tattva, also known as the element of fire and join it with the Prithvi Tattva, which is Earth element. The mantra for Agni Bija means "ram."

1. Keep the left nostril in close take a deep breath via the nose of your left. Then mentally repeat "ram" sixteen times.

2. Take a deep breath, then be aware of your mind and "ram" 64 times.

3. Close your right nostril and let your breath go through your left nostril while mentally repeating "ram" 32 times.

Look up to the point of your nose, and think about the bright reflection of the moon's light while you chant"tham" the bija phrase "tham."

1. Keep the right nostril in place and breathe through the left nostril , mentally repeating "tham" sixteen times.

2. Take a deep breath, and then think about chanting "tham" 64 times.

3. Take the left nostril in and breathe out the right nostril, while mentally singing "tham" 32 times.

When you've completed these three pranayamas your nadis is purified. If you find it difficult to master, don't worry about it. It's possible to work towards it.

Bhastrika

If you feel sluggish Don't look for that 5th cup of coffee. Instead, do your breathing routine. Bhastrika is also known as "bellows breath" assists in increasing your prana flow. Many people utilize this technique to increase their energy as well as to calm an over-active mind. If you feel hazy or struggling through the water, Bhastrika can help clear the fog. It is regarded as a warming breathing method that mimics the fanning of an open flame.

The name refers to the active in the filling and emptying stomach and lungs during the exercise. It assists in igniting the fire within your mind and body and aids in digestion. It helps balance Vata and Kapha However, it is important to use it with caution in case pitta becomes irritated.

Bellows breathing is also beneficial in order to lose some weight. A few times of this every day will improve your digestive power and improve your metabolism. It is not recommended to perform this breathing exercise right before bedtime or within a few hours after waking, since it may stimulate your mind and lead to difficulty falling asleep. If you're in need of an energy boost you can try this. The other benefits of this breathing method include:

* Enhances vitality and vigor within the mind and body.

* Helps to create a sense of calm, focus and serenity

* Balances and strengthens the nervous system.

* Supports proper elimination

* Increases circulation

* Purifies your nasal passages and chest and sinuses of mucus.

* Helps to alleviate asthma and allergies.

* Rejuvenates and cleans the liver, spleen and the pancreas

* Kindle's digestive fire can tone the digestive system.

* Aids in the elimination of carbon dioxide

* Infuses blood with oxygen

* It strengthens the heart and lungs.

* Tone abdominal muscles diaphragm and diaphragm as well as the bronchial and the heart

* Increases lung capacity

* Cleans and rejuvinates the lung.

* Toxins are burned off

119

* Balances that are not paid Kapha, Vata, and pitta

This is an advanced practice, and you should be sure that you're comfortable in abdominal breathing. The directions are designed to provide a safeand general introduction to the breathing technique.

To perform Bellows Breath:

1. Choose a comfortable position. The position of sitting cross-legged is ideal, with an ottoman or blanket to help raise the hips. You can also relax in a chair, with your feet laid flat.

2. Be sure to sit straight with your shoulders relaxed. Inhale deeply via your nostrils. Relax your hands upon your knees. Every time you exhale take a deep breath, let your belly expand completely. The eyes should close when you feel at ease doing it.

3. It is possible to begin by doing the full yoga breathing cycle that we discussed earlier to activate the prana maya Kosha.

4. For your first bhastrika start by taking an inhale by using the full yoga breathing method. Then, take a long exhale, without

pressure or stress. While exhaling then let your stomach expand and contract by pulling the belly button toward the spine, as the diaphragm expands toward the lung.

5. This exhale should be followed by a powerful inhale without tension or tension or. Inhale and let your stomach expand and expand by pulling off the stomach button from your spine. Let diaphragms drop to the lower pelvis floor.

6. Then, take another powerful exhale. Keep your attention on your breath as you breathe both in and out, making sure that the length of the breaths the same.

7. It is important to ensure that your breath is controlled and comes through your diaphragm. You should ensure that your shoulders neck, chest, and head are still, and the only thing that moves is your belly.

The first session should consist of 10 cycles. When you've reached the tenth round, you should stop and resume your normal breathing, paying attention to any sensations that you feel in your body or your mind. You should give yourself 15 to 30 minutes of breathing normally and then begin the next session. The next round will take 20 breaths. Stop after 30 secs of normal breathing. Then, do one final cycle of 30 breaths.

If you'd like to include the power of hand position during your training, prior to you start your bellows breath create a fist using your hands and place your hands close to your shoulders.

When you are first beginning to learn this, you should keep your breathing moderately slow, but powerful. Try to take a breath every 2 seconds. Make sure you take a break between each round. As you continue to training, your ab muscles will get stronger which will allow you to increase your practice the number of rounds to 5.

Be aware of your body while doing this. Bellows breathing is safe however, if you begin feeling lightheaded, stop for a few seconds and breathe in a natural way. If the discomfort is gone you can try a second round however, keep it slow and less invigorating.

Breath exercises should be done when you first awake. As this can help in reviving your body performing this exercise as the first step will help to wake your body and increase blood flow.

It is also a great tool to get you through the midday slump. The midday slump usually occurs just after lunch, making it hard to get through the rest of your day. Find a quiet spot that isn't crowded and try several breaths of bellows to get you going instead of having an coffee.

It is also a good breathing exercise to do prior to a exercise. It helps to relax your body and get you focused on your work.

Avoid this breathing technique if are pregnant or going through menstrual cycles. If you suffer from seizures that are not controlled, panic disorder epilepsy, hypertension or suffer from glaucoma, nosebleeds or detached retina or recent abdominal surgery. It is not advisable to do this when you've just consumed food.

Dosha-Changing Pranayamas

Every pranayama practice has an impact on the body-mind system. Ayurveda will teach you which types of exercises are suitable for different individuals. Nadi Shodana, also referred to as alternate nostril breathing allows you to breathe alternately through your right and left nostrils. It has a direct link with your brain. The left nostril, it affects the right hemisphere of the brain and the right nostril is connected to the left.

Everyone has nostril dominance which means we mainly breathe through our noses. But throughout the day, this dominance may shift. Pranayama can aid in balancing this, but it's the reason why it is important to align your Dosha.

The following habits will impact your dosha. There are three types of doshas: Vata, Kapha, and pitta. These are energy types that are present throughout us and we all have a predominant dosha kind.

Pitta is a fierce and fiery kind of person who will appreciate a power trip every now and then. They can eat an entire mountain of food, and they are prepared to eat another meal within a few hours.

Veta is an incredibly delicate species and is unable to warm up. They might eat, graze or snack through the day, but often find themselves in need of take a break. They also love engaging in conversation about a range of subjects and are likely to repeat their thoughts several times.

Kapha is a happy person and, with a lot of thought take three bites of cake. They loved to be sitting on the couch calling loved ones, offering positive and encouraging tips.

Doshas play an active role in your life, constantly changing in response to conditions like weather, stress, or the conditions. Your habits, whether good or not, are triggered due to your doshas. You might be prone to eat too much ice cream or spend too much time on phones, or not sleep when you require it most. Your lifestyle choices can impact your life in either positive or negative ways.

Through the pranayama methods listed below You can even out or switch your dosha as you require.

Surya Bhedana

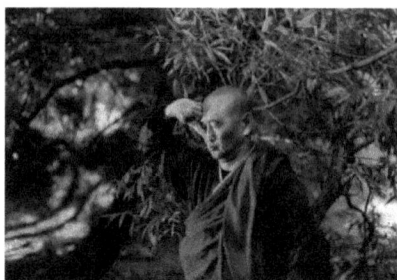

Surya Bhedana is a warm pranayam that focuses at the left nostril. Surya which means sun, refers to the right nostril. The nostril that is located there is connected with the Pingala nodi. Bhedana refers to passing through or to pierce. If you shut your nostril and force prana to go through only one side, you'll experience a warming effect within the body. This could help correct the imbalance in coolness which is normal in vata and/or Kapha dosha.

The typical person will experience a clash between their cooling and warming energies, which can lead to illness. This breath works with Chandra Bhedana, which we will discuss in the next section to aid in balancing the body.

1. Begin by finding the position of sitting comfortably in order to ensure your neck and spine are in alignment.

2. Let your eyes close and focus your attention on your eye's third, which is located in the area between your eyebrows.

3. Take a moment to observe your breathing and take the time to take a deep breath for a few times and allow your lungs to fillup while expanding your abdominal during the inhaleand contracting as you exhale.

4. Relax your left arm on your lap or by your side. Use the right hand and then use the ring finger to stop the left nostril from opening. The two fingers you are using should be folded in your palm.

5. Breathe deeply and slowly by using the right nostril only.

6. Keep your breath in for a few seconds. If you suffer from hypertension or hypertension, or both don't hold your breath for long.

7. The left nostril should be opened and close the right one using the thumb. Then slowly exhale.

8. Repeat breathing in through your right nostril and out via the left side for between one and three minutes.

9. After you've finished take your left arm to rest on your lap or by your side and take a few deep breaths before you open your eyes.

If you suffer from an issue with blood pressure or heart disease, you might prefer to avoid this exercise. If you are planning to use Surya Bhedana as well as Chandra Bhedana, you should not do both at the same time.

Chandra Bhedana

Chandra is the reverse of Surya. Chandra means moon. Left nostrils are utilized for breath in and the right for exhaling. When you practice this breathing the energy flows via to the Ida Nadi. This is linked to the cooling aspect of the body, and also stimulates the parasympathetic nervous systems.

Practicing Chandra Bhedana helps to reduce body heat. It is beneficial for those who have high blood pressure. It helps lower fevers. It assists in stabilizing the mind and ease tension, stress and other mental issues.

1. Begin by settling into a comfortable sitting in a comfortable seated. You'll want your spine and neck aligned and your torso to be free so that you are able to breathe.

2. It is recommended to use your left hand to practice this and hold it as you did during Surya Bhandana, with the middle and index fingers folded over the palm, with the thumb just below the left nostril and the ring fingers just to the right.

3. Before beginning, you should choose the inhale, hold and exhale ratio. In the classic yoga texts they recommend using the ratio 1:4:2. This could be as simple as inhaling for two seconds and holding for 8 seconds, and then breathing out for 4 seconds. For newbies, it's recommended that you adhere with a 1:1 proportion, and do not hold for too long.

4. Close your eyes before you start your exercise.

5. With the ring finger, shut the right nostril, then take a deep breath.

6. Keep your breath in for a few seconds, then, open your right nostril, and close the

left nostril with your thumb. Relax your breath slowly and gradually.

7. Repeat this procedure for anywhere from one or two minutes.

Do not practice Chandra Bhedana during the winter cold months or if you suffer from a cold as it can enhance the body's cooling. People who suffer from epilepsy or have low blood pressure should be careful when they decide to do this.

Shitali

Shitali is sometimes spelled sheetali, is referred to for its cooling effect. This is a breathing exercise which helps cool the body, emotions and mind. It is derived from it being the Sanskrit term sheet which means "frigid" as well as "cold." Sheetal translates to "that that is peaceful and calming, without passion, and relaxing." This practice assists in calming and relax the mind-body connection through activating an evaporative cooling mechanism as you breathe. It delivers a cooling, gentle energy to the tissues of your body. Incredibly, this method will also ignite the digestive fire, much as a piece of coal that has been coated with ash could begin to glow in the presence of a cool gush of wind.

Shitali is a great practice to do in situations of the heat, experiencing an emotional crisis that is heated hot flashes, extended exposure to sunlight and intense physical activity or other situations that can cause heat. It is a balanced practice for pitta, and is neutral towards Kapha or Vata. However, it is important to be careful when practicing this when you are suffering from an excess of cold in your body or are experiencing particularly cold weather. In this case it is important to determine which shitali practice is the most effective pranayama to be practicing right now. If it is, think about mixing this practice into heating pranayama like Bhastrika.

The benefits of shitali include:

Reduces blood pressure

* Quenchs thirsty excess

* Alleviates excess hunger

* Enhances immunity

* Sooths colicky pain

* Reducing fever

* Helps to create a sense of satisfaction

* Increases prana flow within the body

* Calms and soothes the mind, promoting peace of mind.

* Helps reduce inflammation

* Helps soothe skin inflammation

* Relieves hyper acidity within the digestive tract.

* Kindles are a digestive fire that helps improve digestion

The body is cooled, and gets rid of heat.

* Balances excess pitta

Before beginning the practice, shitali asks for you to roll up your tongue in a circular motion by rolling the edges upwards to form the shape of a tube. If you're unable to accomplish this, there's another variant of this called sitkari. We'll discuss that in the next section.

Patients suffering from respiratory conditions such as bronchitis, excessive mucus or asthma, and people with poor blood pressure must steer clear of this method of elimination. Constipated people may be advised to stay clear of this practice too. Patients with heart diseases may do this, but do not do the breath retention. Because the method requires inhaling through your mouth, which does not remove things such as the nasal passages, you must refrain from doing heavy environmental polluting.

1. Similar to other techniques of pranayama it is best to practice this with a full stomach. Come into a comfortable seated position. A cross-legged position on the floor with your legs elevated slightly using an extra blanket or pillow is ideal. If you're not comfortable sitting in a chair. Just ensure that you ensure your feet are flat in the dirt.

2. Relax your hands into contact with your knees and then let your spine stretch to ensure that your neck, head and back are straight while keeping your chest and abdomen erect.

3. Relax your eyes and breathe through your nose.

4. Relax your body and then do several rounds of deep yoga breathing.

5. When you're ready begin to take the cool breath.

6. Take your tongue out and curl the edges to create the shape of a tube. Breathe through your tongue curled as if you breathed into straws.

7. When you breathe in, breathe exactly similar to an entire yogic breath. inhaling into the middle-section of the lower abdominal and chest. You will notice how cool the effect of air.

8. When you are at the peak of your breath, draw your tongue back into your mouth then close your mouth and then keep your breath for a couple of seconds. A few seconds are sufficient. You can increase the length of the time you keep your breath.

9. After that, slowly let the breath go through your nose. This is one breath of cooling.

You can do this for seven times. If you'd like to do more time to practice, slowly increase the number of rounds fifteen rounds. When you are at a point where you are ready to bring your workout at an end take a moment of relaxation and breathe out and in with your mouth. Your breath will return to normal. You can take a moment to notice the way you feel. What are you feeling physically? Are you feeling cooler? What are the sensations you experience? Take a moment to observe your thoughts and thoughts. Once you're at peace to go about your day, take your eyes off and pay attention to the world surrounding you.

Sitkari

Sitkari practice is the identical pranayama technique like shitaki, but it's modified to accommodate those who cannot roll their tongues. Around a third of the population are genetically ineligible to roll their tongues into tubes. Sitkari refers to "hiss" also known as "sip." If you follow this technique, you'll have to breathe in your mouth using closed teeth. This can produce a hissing sound. The benefits of sittingkari are similar to those mentioned above in the rest of the routine.

Follow the steps previously mentioned until you reach the point where you are instructed for you to make your tongue curl. Instead, extend your tongue and then flatten it. Carefully place your tongue between your teeth, allowing the lips move apart and then widen slightly as if smiling. Inhale and let your breath flow across the tongue's sides and into your mouth.

Continue to follow the steps above, and complete seven sitkari breaths in a row.

The same guidelines for sitali must be taken into consideration for the sitkari, too. It's also important to make sure the breath you're taking in is similar to your the body temperature as your nostrils aren't going to be able to warm your breath. So if you're outdoors and it's very cold, you should not to inhale that air as it may cause irritation to your lung.

Ujjayi Kumbhaka

This ujjayi pranayama practice is a great way to ease tension in the mind as well as help to warm your body. By doing this it is possible to complete filling your lungs with air as you relax your throat and breathe through your nose. This breathing technique which is often used in vinyasa as well as ashtanga yoga exercises.

It's derived directly from it's Sanskrit word ujjayi which means "to become victorious" or "to overcome." It is the reason why it is sometimes as "victorious breath." If done properly, it produces sounds similar to the sway of waves in the ocean, hence the other name "ocean breath."

The ability to maintain a steady, consistent breathing is among the most essential aspects of yoga. If you can control your breathing it will help you calm your mind and draw focus to the present moment. This kind of mindfulness is at the core of yoga. Yoga is an instruction that, when you practice breathing with conscious control, you will create positive changes in your emotional, spiritual physical and mental health.

Contrary to many other pranayamas that can be performed sitting or lying down Ujjayi is typically performed during your yoga practice during every pose. The sound, depth and steadyness that comes from the ujjayi breath can help to connect your mind, spirit and body to the present. This fusion will add an additional dimension and depth for your practice of yoga.

If you regularly practice ujjayi you will be able to release any tension. The increased oxygen levels and the deep exhalations will boost and energize the physical training. It can help to calm your mind. It is also beneficial to people suffering from insomnia, tension in the mind or anxiety. Over time, you'll discover the best method to direct your breath so that it can be the guide for your practice.

When you are practicing ujjayi, ensure that you don't strain the throat. Be careful if have respiratory problems such as asthma or emphysema. Make sure to stop immediately if you are feeling faint or dizzy. Make sure you're always in control of your abilities and limitations, and do not over-exert yourself to the limit. These techniques are intended to benefit but not cause harm to you. If you are concerned regarding your health, consult your doctor prior to using this.

Begin by finding an upright position. Relax your body and let your eyes shut. Relax your jaw to down a little, and let your jaw and tongue relax.

Breathe in and breathe out with your mouth. Feel the air moving through your mouth as you breathe into.

When you breathe out then gently press the back of your throat, similar to what the way you speak when you talk. Slightly whisper "ahh," as you exhale. If you want to help to imagine you're trying to block the window.

When you are more comfortable with the way your exhale is feeling, you can maintain your breathing in a constricted manner. in. Soon, you will begin hearing your breathing make sounds like ocean.

When you are in with your breathing control, allow your mouth close , and take your breath only through the nose. Keep the same tightness in your throat that you experienced when you had your mouth wide. You should be able in the direction of hearing. Your breath should be directed towards the vocal cords and towards the lower back of your throat. The mouth should remain shut with your lips relaxed.

Focus on the breath. Allow this sound to calm the mind. It should be possible to be able to hear the breath, but someone who is standing a few feet away from you should not be able listen to it.

Be sure that your inhalations are completely filled with air and completely release the air as you exhale.

Practice this for 5 minutes. Then, you can extend the time by 15 mins. It is possible to begin linking your breathing to your movements slowly. When you practice ujjayi when you do asanas, breathe in while you stretch and expand while exhaling when you fold and stretch.

The most frequently made mistake by this breath is tightening the throat. It should be only the slightest constriction. Once you are more comfortable with this, you will be able to utilize it throughout every yoga class without stopping. You may also seek out your yoga instructor for comments on whether you're following the correct procedure or require modifications. For advanced practitioners, you can try different variations, but with the proper guidance. Bandhas are also a possibility, or muscular locks, such as those used to lock the throat, but only after you've practiced it enough.

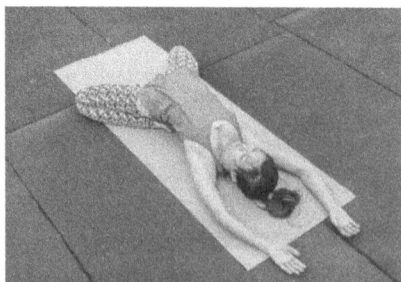

Kapalbhati

Kapalbhati is considered an intermediate-advanced practice made up of powerful and short exhales followed by a passive inhale. The intention behind this practice is to cleanse your body, and to help to cleanse and tone the respiratory system. This is accomplished by stimulating your body to eliminate the toxins and waste. This can leave your body and mind feeling refreshed and rejuvenated.

If you practice pranayama regularly the majority of your toxins are eliminated by exhaling. The practice of regularly kapalbhati aids in detoxifying the body. The most obvious indicator of being healthy is having a glowing forehead.

The broken down kapalbhati can be described as two Sanskrit words "kapala," meaning skull as well as "bhati," meaning light. This is why it's often referred to as "skull lightener breath" as well as "light respiration of the skull." While you practice this, it is possible to imagine the area around your skull being filled with the light of the enlightenment. It is likely that you have experienced"the breath of fire and that is the reason for this practice.

Kapalabhati is a warming and invigorating. It purifies your respiratory tract, lungs and sinuses, helping to help prevent the occurrence of allergies and other illnesses. It is a good habit to regularly practice this exercise and helps strengthen abdominal muscles and the diaphragm. This exercise will also help improve your blood flow, boost your energy levels and stimulate your brain helping you to get prepared for your meditation, and any other activity that requires your attention. Other benefits include:

* Calms and uplifts the mind.

It stimulates the nervous system, and also helps recharge the brain.

* It can help to trim and tighten the belly.

* Enhances the digestive tract's functioning assimilation, absorption, and digestion of nutrients

* Enhances blood circulation and gives an extra glow to the face.

* Stimulates abdominal organs, making it useful for people who suffer from diabetes.

* Removes the Nadis

* It increases your metabolism helping you lose weight

Kapalabhati is a sophisticated technique. Do not attempt this if you're not proficient in breathing techniques that are basic. Avoid doing this if suffer from heart disease, hernia and/or hypertension. Women who are pregnant should not do this as well. Take care when tackling this in case you have any type of respiratory problem, such as asthma or emphysema.

It is best to stop exercising when you begin to feel faint or dizzy. Be sure to work within your capabilities and limitations.

1. To begin, you must get into a comfortable in a position that allows you to maintain your spine in a straight line and your stomach free. In case sitting down on the ground is not a good choice for you then you could also be seated in a chair. Just ensure that you remain on your feet on the ground and your back straight.

2. Let your hands rest sitting on the floor.

3. Focus your attention on your lower abdomen. It is also possible to place the palms of your hands one on top of the other, over the lower part of your abdomen.

4. Breathe deeply by putting your nose in.

5. Engage the lower abdomen. You can also apply your hands and push into the abdomen, pushing the breath to come out of a quick blast.

6. Let this contraction go quickly, allowing an inhale that is automatic and passive. It is important to keep your attention solely on the exhale. The rest will remain in unfocused.

7. Begin slowly, striving for 65-70 contractions per minute. Gradually increase the pace so that you are able to achieve 95-105 cycles per minute. Be sure to stick to your own pace and never stop if begin to feel faint or dizzy.

8. After about a minute taking the time to breathe deeply through your nose, and then take a breath out slowly through your mouth. Depending on how proficient the technique is, could repeat the process for a second round.

If you do this exercise properly, you'll start feeling energized, revitalized and clean. It requires familiarity and understanding of the basics of the methods. Be sure, if have never tried this practice, to become familiar with ujjayi. It will also be beneficial to keep in mind the following tips while doing this:

* If your breathing ever becomes strained, or you get dizzy or anxious then stop and breathe in a regular manner.

* Do not push your breath to either the exhale or the inhale.

Make sure your spine and shoulders in a straight line while doing this exercise. The only thing you should be moving is your lower belly.

Your abdomen should not be contracted while you breathe.

Focus on your abdomen's lower part, and exhale.

Other precautions to take for this technique of pranayama are those with an artificial pacemaker or stent back pain caused by a slip disc, hernia or epilepsy, or who have recently undergone abdominal surgery. Women should not practice this when they are pregnant, just had a baby and are in menstrual cycles.

Sama Vritti

Sama Vritti pranayama can be translated to equal or similar variations. If practiced it requires a constant exhale and an inhale of the same length. This breathing pattern assists in relaxing your body and mind. If you feel stressed, disoriented, stressed in a state of overwhelm, this breathing pattern helps you assist and maintain the steady change in your parasympathetic nervous system. It is a great way to calm and calm an hyperactive Vata to ensure that your body and mind can rest.

Sama vritti is a popular choice in the practice of asana. If you can master this while sitting and you'll increase the flow of your movements while maintaining a stronger connection and steady breathing.

Begin by settling into a comfortable, seated posture with your hips raised by a pillow or blanket. It is possible to sit in a chair, and keep your feet to the ground. This can help to support your diaphragm and allow breathing to flow smoothly. It is also possible to practice this when lying down.

Once you've settled, you can begin to notice the natural breathing patterns you are accustomed to. Note how long your breaths last and the feelings that you feel throughout your body. Pay attention to how you transition between your inhale and your exhale. If you are feeling tension, consider how you can alter it to ease it and let go of tension in the transitions.

* Now begin counting on the inhale. Breathe deeply in for four times. Inhale and breathe out for a count of four. Repeat for a few times.

* If the number of four is too low it is possible to slowly begin increasing the count, gradually increasing it to 10. The key is to ensure that the count is identical for both the exhale and inhale. Maintain your count to a level that you find comfortable.

* Try 10 rounds of this breath at an easy pace. Keep letting your mind relax and remain in the present. If you lose the count, begin with a fresh start.

* When you finish your practice and bring it to an end, let your breath to return to normal. Note any changes you notice in your body or mind.

It is possible to add retentions on the top of your breath, and hold them for the same amount of time as breathing out and in. If you're not used to this practice, you may remove the retentions in case they feel uncomfortable. It is also possible to keep your retentions shorter if have to. It's important to ensure to ensure that the breath you take both in and out remains identical.

Do not overdo it or push your breath while performing these or other types of pranayama method. If you're pregnant it is possible to practice this breathing technique, but take a break from the retentions. For those with ear, eye or heart issues or with high blood pressure should not hold their breath. If you suffer from lower blood pressure do not hold your breath following the exhale.

There are a variety of other pranayama practices, however those are by far the most widely practiced and come with many advantages. For those who are new to pranayama, take it slowly and begin with basic methods until you are accustomed to the sensation of deep belly breathes.

Chapter 14: The Yogi's Diet

Yoga also offers suggestions for your daily life like the way you eat and how you sex. This section will cover several important lifestyle choices you must consider in order to live a the most healthy lifestyle.

Sexuality and the way it impacts Your Life

In our modern times and especially in the West When someone thinks of yoga and sexuality typically conjures images of celibate monks strutting around wearing orange clothes. They might also think of the opposite of this and that would be sexual sex that claims to promise its users the highest levels of consciousness, however this could be somewhat awry to certain. What do yoga's teachings actually say about sexuality?

According to yoga, sexual sex is an act of worship that involves two souls who merge and merge into one. It's an experience that isn't normal, in which our souls transcend and dance with the opposites and finally become one as in Tantra. It is among the closest experiences you'll be able to experience infinity.

If you search for "sex" within the Dictionary, you could see a definition which says something like "sexual union which involved the penetration of vaginal tissue with penis." This defines sexual relations as physical however it does not include all of the above. It's just basic sex.

Sex is the Greek root, which translates to "separation," which reinforces the difference between two people. Yoga is the total opposite of the word "sex. The meaning of yoga is "to remove the separation, or to tie." Yoga is considered to be an Tantric practice. Tantra is an Sanskrit word which simply translates to"to "tan" which means to stretch, and "tra" over. It is believed that the English words for traverse and travel originate out of the exact same word "tra." Tantra is actually about the ability to expand your perspective of yourself and others or even to cross the gap that separates individuals from one another.

The Patanjali sutras, one can learn how sexual energy can be extremely powerful. When it is directed to the higher Chakras this can result in a more spiritual level of consciousness. Semen is also known in the form of "ojas," and it was never intended to be thrown away. Semen doesn't only function as a sexy fluid but also a lubricant for brain and nervous system. According to yoga theory that require eighty bites of food for the smallest drop of blood and the blood of 80 drops makes one drop of semen.

In the West the majority of people's views regarding yoga were influenced by Shankaracharya, who was a teacher of Vedanta in the 8th century and led the movement known as the Sannyasin. The monks who were celibate and wore orange robes and were averse to the practices that were prevalent in the modern world. A different teacher in 1550, Vallabhacharya, taught people that the only way to get to God was through worldly activities. The people in the lineage of Vallabhacharya were married. Monks were striving to attain the higher levels of being.

In the Hatha Yoga Pradipika and the Patanjali's Yoga Sutra, Yoga didn't hold a negative view of the world. But, it does state that yoga views uninformed minds or a body that is not cleansed as a hurdle that could hinder them from achieving an enlightened state.

Yoga can help a person to work on their body and mind to cleanse their bodies and conquer all bad, old, and karmic habits. Yoga transforms the body into a tool that can be utilized to gain access to or greater knowledge that can enable the moksha-liberation process out of samsara as well as the cycle that is life, birth, and death.

The Yogi Bhajan instructed his students that they only need to take a break once per month. You read it exactly. He also said that it is vital to maintain the man's "ojas." When it can be done, it is possible to increase his Kundalini energy. He also stated that sexual activity starts three days before you actually engage in sexual relations. This was what was once known by the name of "courtship." This was recommended for the woman to have a location that she felt safe and secure. It is also a good place for couples can rest after the event. It is possible to get the space set up in her honor by lighting candles or using scent therapy and any other thing you can think will ensure that her body and mind are at relaxed.

Sexual experiences of a person are able to be engraved in their subconscious mind and aura. Each one will be interspersed with different intensity. A too-intense flirt could cause holes in your appearance as well.

Bhajan's teachings state the female body has two lines of arc. The first line is a line that runs between one and the next and is referred to as the Halo. The color of this one will depend on their physical and mental health. The others are moving from nipple to. The first one is engraved with the many sexual experiences they've experienced in their lives. Women must clear these energy fields to keep their body clear and strong.

Women's energy is very sensitive. Electromagnetic fields have an extremely destructive impact on their. They can cause them to be very fragile emotionally. If the relationships she has with her family are built on trust, respect as well as love, then she will prosper and be awe-inspiring and secure, vibrant and creative.

An individual's intent will affect the outcome of any action. If you're looking to cleanse your actions, then you need to be able to express your intentions in a clear manner. One could decide to engage in sexual sex because of motives that are not their own, like trying to get the upper hand or to humiliate their partner. Someone else is having sexual relations with someone else to lift them up and appreciate their partner. There are some who would describe the first in terms of "rape," whereas the second is to be "making the decision to love." Both are the same thing, but they were each performed with different motives.

Consider for a few minutes about the time we use in our lives, whether unconsciously or conscious because of sex, our clothes or behave, our purchasing choices, our sexual desires, how we appear at our appearance, and many more.

Spend a few minutes and reflect on the way your life could be different without sex present. You may be surprised by the significant role that sexuality plays in your daily life.

Sexuality and religion used to be a pair However, spiritual practices have become more prevalent in every way and more and more people are bringing meaning to their sexual encounters. Sexual intimacy is a beautiful combination, but it can be a sacred experience too.

Let's return to Tantric sexual relations for a second. The principal purpose for Tantra is to provide two people with faces, so that they can view the other as individuals. If you gaze into the eyes of another and look into their eyes, you'll be able to see yourself. This is the primary practice of yoga. It is also known as shunyata or emptyness. It basically means that everyone that we meet actually comes from us. We could call them the essences that come up from our previous Karma. If you're in a relationship with someone else, and you decided to examine their eyes, or to be completely naked and I'm certainly not speaking about being physically naked but also spiritually naked, it may make you feel uncomfortable in the present.

One benefit of Tantric sexual activity is the ability to cleanse your subconscious. In the course of treatment the memories of painful or traumatic events may surface, and people may experience emotional highs and lows. It is possible that they are feeling content, but then they feel sad and starts crying, and aren't sure what caused it. Once you know the reason for this and you understand why, you will see your spouse in new perspective.

Love can be a scary thing. If you're in love, there's not any other people or faces since you are one body. In the vastness of there's not a lot of space for human bodies which is the reason the majority of people engage in sexual sex to have fun.

There is a possibility of achieving enlightened sex however it is very uncommon. If you're looking to attain enlightenment and enlightenment, celibacy is the best choice. Celibacy should not be encouraged when it's not your personal choice. If you take this decision simply because someone else told you it's the right choice or that it makes you holy and pure It will result in suffering and trouble and will not ever last.

Brahmacharya which could be translated as celibacy, is a method that Patanjali suggests. For many that means you need to avoid sexual contact. Brahma is a reference to God Charya is a reference to a vehicle that could be used to travel, thus brahmacharya refers to "to engage in sexual activity with the intent of moving towards God." It is possible to modify it as "moving towards Yoga."

The way we view sexuality today is a result of when we started domesticating animals, which meant breeding them, and possibly having the ability to control them sexually. Animal industries do not think of the animals in relation to their health or happiness. They are viewed as objects that can be abused sexually, and later taken away for food.

The connection between sexual sexual assault and murder should inform that you everything you must learn about our way of living. If the bulk of our economy is built on sexually abusing animals and then killing them for profit This affects how our intimate relationships with fellow humans. If you don't have a connection then you're not going to enjoy any intimacy.

Sexuality is compartmentalized by humans as an additional function or a obligation that we are required to perform, and the majority times it is done without compassion or love. We are told that our bodies are distinct from our mind and spirit. This means that we've separated our spirituality from our physical body.

What can we do to transform sexual intimacy from being made to be exploited, and instead see an individual as something beyond their genitalia and the things they could do for us? The first step is to ask: "What can they do for me?" We have to change the question to: "What could I do to help my partner?" "Is there a way to enhance their lives?" "What could I do to make them feel more loved, appreciated and more happy, or even better?"

All it takes is staring them in the eye and askingthem "Who is this person?" "Who am I?" "Who are we?" "What are we doing?" "Why are we doing this?" All of these are extremely relevant questions.

Everything that we see around us reflect the reality in us all. Yoga is a way to connect and sex could be one of separation. Yoga lets you look at yourself as other people. It allows you to feel them so much that they disappear and you merge into one. If this happens, sex disappears however the love remains. This is the reason why love is so important.

What You Must Eat Well

Our physical and mental health is influenced by the foods we consume, the manner in which we eat, and also the quantity of food we consume. Mitahara is among the Yamas in the old Indian practices. Mita simply refers to "moderate," and ahara is "diet." In other words, to simplify, mitahara would mean to take a moderately balanced diet.

It is advised to consume food only when you feel hungry. If you are able to see sweet foods It isn't necessarily referring to food items that are sugary, it is a reference to pleasant taste, fresh, and fresh foods. The act of offering a portion of your food to Shiva signifies that you should consume food that will nourish your body in order to become an instrument of spirituality.

Yoga doesn't categorize foods into categories like proteins, fats and carbohydrates. They are placed in groups such as Taamsik Raajsik and Saatvic in accordance with their effects on the body and mind. Tamasic foods cause you to feel tired or fatigued. Raajsik foods can cause energy and a sense of rest. Sattvic food will make you feel energetic as well as energetic and easy.

Certain foods should avoid at all times. They are referred to as Apathy. There are certain foods can be eaten, which are known as Pathya.

It's not healthy to consume food items that were heated after they've cooled. It's not a good idea to consume food items that do not contain any natural oils or are dried. It's not a good idea to consume food items that are acidic, salty or old.

A balanced diet should include purified water, some fruits such as cucumbers, dry ginger honey, crystallized sugar brown sugar, ghee milk, barley, wheat, rice and cereals.

The most significant thing to remember about eating a healthy diet is that it has to feed seven dhatus: semen or ova as well as fat, marrow blood, bone, flesh and the skin. Foods that disrupt the body's balance naturally shouldn't be consumed.

The best kinds of food isn't all needed. It is important to understand what amount of food we should consume and the right time to eat it. Our bodies will determine when we've reached the maximum amount of food we can consume. If we be attentive to our bodies and begin to eat mindfully and mindfully, we'll know when it is time to stop eating. It is not a good idea to spend Prana to digest.

A relaxed and happy attitude when cooking and eating can aid in keeping Prana into your meal. You should not take in too much or eat too small. It is not advisable to rest too much or too excessively.

Yoga is a method of practice which can bring your mind and body to one another and stop thoughts that wander around. Diet is an integral part of the human experience and yoga is a way to do this. When discussing Indian philosophical thought the diet is believed to be an esoteric entity. One grows through the food they eat. Shrimadbhagvad Gita defines a healthy diet to be well-balanced.

A diet that fully encompasses Yoga practices is known as an Yogic diet. According to their doctrine, the majority of the food we consume provide nourishment to the skin while the subtle elements of food are nourishing the other organs of our body. If you are looking to increase your consciousness, you must to cleanse your outer sheath with the prescribed diet outlined within Yogic Scriptures. These texts speak about the timing, quantity, quality, as well as the sequence to eat food.

Diet plays a crucial aspect in the success you achieve when exercising Yoga. If you wish to achieve success, you must start by choosing the appropriate food items. Consuming the right food is important prior to practicing pranayama.

If you are practicing yoga without managing your diet, you'll be suffering from various illnesses and will not progress. If your food and fun are in balance Your movements and actions will be in harmony Your sleeping and waking will be in harmony and your practice will relieve all your troubles.

There are three kinds of diets: Tamasic, Rajasic, and Sattvic. Everyone has three characteristics that determine the preferences and preferences of others. The people who possess three characteristics are likely to have three different food preferences. The Shri Krishna puts their diet in three categories.

Tamasic Diet

The foods in this diet can be very heavy and result in fatigue or lethargy. These food items should avoid at all cost especially those suffering from depression or a chronic disease. Tamasic foods are unripe fruits or overripe fruits food items that are rotten and stale food items alcohol the red meat of processed food deep-fried food items, burnt foods, or foods that are fermented.

Rajasic Diet

They should be stayed away from, and include: any caffeinated beverage, excessively processed food items, artificial additives food items, spicy, foods that cause irritation to mucus membranes of the body, mushrooms onion and garlic, among others.

Sattvic Diet

The diet is based on foods in their natural state. Fresh foods that do not contain any preservatives or additives. These are foods that should be consumed in their natural in any way that is feasible, like fresh, cooked lightly or steaming. This diet is comprised of fresh fruits and vegetables whole grains as well as lentils, nuts, pulses, seeds natural sweeteners such as honey, and spices.

Quality of Sleep

Sleep is vital for health and well-being However, millions of people do not get enough of rest, and the majority of them suffer from this. Certain studies have found that over 40 million Americans suffer from 70 different sleep disorders. In addition, 60% of the adults who were surveyed said they had trouble sleeping for only a couple of times per week.

Many of them went untreated and have not been diagnosed. More than 40 percent of adults who are asked to admit they have a problem with sleep that is so bad that it affects their lives. Around 69 percent of kids have had sleep issues at least once a week.

Sleeping is as important as eating a healthy , balanced diet and exercising regularly. The modern world doesn't always acknowledge the need to sleeping, but it's equally important to our overall health. It is essential to take the effort to get regular, uninterrupted sleep. Here are some advantages that come when we get enough sleep:

More Concentration and Productivity

A variety of studies have been conducted to study the effects that the effects of sleep deprivation on our bodies. The researchers concluded that sleep is linked to certain brain functions for example:

* Cognition

* Productivity

* Concentration

A study from 2015 revealed that sleep patterns of children could affect their academic performance as well as their behavior.

Low Weight Gain

There is an association between sleep patterns, obesity or weight gain however it's not entirely certain. There have been numerous studies that have connected inadequate sleep to weight gain.

Another study done recently states that there's not any link between sleeping insufficientness and overweight. The research suggests that previous studies did not consider other variables such as:

* Long sedentary times

* Long working hours

* Educational level

* Physical physical

* Being diagnosed with type 2 diabetes.

* Alcohol consumption

Insufficient sleep can hinder someone's ability or motivation to lead a healthy life However, it may be a factor in weight growth.

Calorie Regulation

It's like weight gain, however this suggests that sleeping enough could allow a person to consume less calories while awake. A study found that sleep patterns can alter a person's hormones that control appetite.

If you're not getting enough sleep this could interfere with your body's ability of regulating the amount of food you consume.

More athletic ability

The National Sleep Foundation says the proper amount of rest for adults should be between seven and nine hours per night. The athletes could benefit from the recommended ten hours of sleep each night. Sleeping is just as important for players as eating the correct quantity of calories and consuming the proper nutrients.

The primary reason for this is that our bodies recover while they sleep. Other benefits could include:

* Mentally functioning better

* Speedier

* More coordination

* Better energy

* Performance improvement

Heart Disease Risk Lowered

The most significant risk factor for developing heart disease is hypertension. The right amount of sleep each night helps our body's blood pressure manage itself. By doing this, you can lower the chance of suffering from conditions like apnea as well as boost overall health of the heart.

More emotional and social intelligence

Some studies also showed that those with sleep problems such as insomnia had more signs of depression.

Lowered Inflammation

A connection has been discovered between adequate sleep and reducing the body's inflammation. A study suggests that there's an association between inflammatory bowel diseases and sleep absence. This study revealed that a lack of sleep was a factor in these conditions and that these conditions may cause sleep loss.

Better Immune System

Sleep can help our bodies recover, regenerate, and repair. It's not just the immune system that's an the only exception. Research has proven that more restful sleep can aid in the fight against diseases. Scientists need to conduct more research in order to determine the precise sleep-related mechanisms that govern the impact it has in our immunity system.

The Signs of Sleep Deprivation

Insomnia, moodiness, and disinhibition are among the first indicators of sleep lack. If you're not getting enough rest after the first small signs, you may start experiencing memory loss multitasking abilities as well as flattened emotional responses slow speech, or being unable to be make the original. If you are beginning to fall to sleep, you could slip into what's known as microsleep . This could cause your attention to drop or they may drift off when reading or driving and later be experiencing hallucinations near the start or end of REM sleep.

Sleep Problems Are the Root of

Stress is the primary factor behind sleep issues. The most common triggers are stress at school or work and marriage or family issues and death or illnesses. The problem usually goes disappear when stress has gone away. If sleep issues, such as insomnia, aren't addressed and they persist, even when the stressor has been eliminated.

Ambient factors such as the temperature of a room, its volume of sound, or levels of brightness can hinder an unrestful sleep. Family members' interruptions or children could disrupt sleeping, too. Be attentive to the dimensions that your mattress is, as well as the quality on your bed, as well as your partner's sleeping habits. If you are sleeping with someone who has a different sleeping preference, who snores, cannot remain asleep, has trouble sleeping, or suffers from another issue, it could quickly become your issue also!

Health Issues

There are a variety of physical ailments that could affect an individual's ability to rest. The conditions that cause pain, such as arthritis, pain or backaches make it difficult to have the rest you need.

Certain studies have suggested that sleep problems that were reported by patient were associated with a higher chance of cardiovascular morbidity and mortality. Women who are pregnant or experiencing changes in hormones could affect sleeptoo.

Certain medicines, including decongestants and steroids as well as treatments for asthma, depression and high blood pressure can produce side effects that could cause insomnia. It's recommended to talk with your physician about any sleep-related issues that persist or last for more than a few weeks.

Many psychiatric conditions can trigger fatigue, such as bipolar disorder or seasonal affective disorder. dysthymia, mixed anxiety-depression minor depression, and postpartum depression.

Sleepiness and Decision Making

In August 2004, researchers conducted research to discover the impact of sleep on risk taking and decision-making. They discovered that lack of sleep can impact the ability to make sound decisions.

Researchers asked for volunteers, and they divided them in two groups. One group was sleep deficient and the other group went to sleep. They were then required to complete a set of tasks using a computer. They were instructed to end their work and collect the money or continue and lose their entire money. If they decided to go on and didn't complete their work within the time allowed the option of losing the entire amount of money.

The people who were more aware felt a sense of compassion for the huge amount of work needed to be completed to complete everything in time and knew the risks that they would lose money. The restless subjects chose to take a break so that they wouldn't be able to lose all their money since they weren't sure they'd be able to complete.

The consequences of sleep deprivation

Many car accidents can be due to people who were sleep deprived. The fact that sleep-deprived drivers have fallen asleep while driving is the cause of 100 000 car accidents, which caused the deaths of 1550 people and injuries to 71,000 per year. Aged 20 or teens were involved in more than 50 percent of the crashes which occur on the roads each year. Lack of sleep may hinder their ability to learn at schools.

A few most likely risk factors for crashes resulting from sleepiness:

* Medical professionals taking a drive home from work

* Night workers

* Drivers of commercial trucks

* Young adult males

* People who receive no more than 6 hours sleep

* Patients with sleepiness that was untreated

• Early in the morning, or at at night driving

Sleep Recommendations

Sleep needs of an individual will differ from one person to the next. It is all dependent on the person's age. As you get older generally, you have less rest for proper functioning.

It is broken into pieces into the following parts:

* 1 until 3 months: 14-17 hours

* 4-12 months * 12 to 16 hours

* 1 to 2 year olds between 11 and 14 hours

3-5 years * 3 to 5 years: 10 to 13 hours

* 6-12 years 9-12 hours

* 13-18 years * 8 to 10 hours

* Between 18 and 60 years 7+ hours

* 61-65 years between 7 and 9 hours

* 65 and over: 7-8 hours

The number of hours isn't so important as the quality of the sleep you're receiving. Here are some indications of poor sleep quality:

* Feeling tired after a long night of sleep

* Waking up numerous times throughout the night

Here are some tips you can try to improve your sleep quality:

* Decrease stress through exercise or therapy

* Get outside and stay active throughout the day.

* You should go to bed every night at the same time.

Do not try to fall asleep after you've had enough rest

Strategies to get Good Sleep

Researchers from the field of sleep believe that the five phases of sleep are defined by the brain waves of an individual which are a reflection of the intensity of sleep or even light sleeping. Sleep in REM is more intense at the beginning of the day. It is during sleep that a person is dreaming and their muscles relax. This is also when your memories are consolidated in your brain.

Experts suggest that hitting the snooze key won't make you feel more rested. It can reduce your rest that you've received. This is due to the fact that it alters the brain's waves. It reduces the REM cycle, which could hinder their mental function throughout the day.

Some techniques can combat sleep problems like:

Try going to bed earlier, for an amount of time. This will ensure that you are getting enough sleep.

* Make the effort of getting up prior to your alarm

* Establish a specific time for bedtime

* Remove any lights, and reduce the sound you hear when you sleep.

* Make sure that the temperature of the room is at a comfortable temperature.

* Do some exercises

* Avoid eating anything weighty before going to the bed

* Do not drink any alcohol-based drinks late into the night.

* Don't smoke if awake in the middle of the night

Do not smoke prior to or when you're getting ready to go to the bed.

* Avoid eating or drinking anything that contains caffeine prior to going to bed.

Create and adhere to an established wake and sleep routine

The importance of sleep is often ignored even when it is an essential aspect of our overall wellbeing and overall health. It is essential to sleep as it aids in the body's repair itself to be well-rested and ready for the following day.

A good amount of rest can help keep us from becoming overweight and ward off heart disease, and reduces the time it takes to recover from disease.

The same applies to the film industry. Many films deal with an obstacle or problem they need to conquer, which includes the usual romantic scene in a restaurant or bedroom. While the film themes may appear similar but all possibilities can be entertaining.

The suggestion that you should control the four urges does not suggest that you need to be immune to these. This doesn't mean you must abstain from them and to live a boring existence. It's a matter of having to manage these impulses in a healthy way to move ahead with your spiritual practice.

Focusing on the Four Areas

There are many other essentials and desires wishes, desires, or needs that are the result of these four. There's a tiny amount in the middle which could make the issue easier to manage. It shouldn't be so difficult to discuss and figure out how to handle this without judgment.

There's a lot of variety in the array of ways that people can manage these four desires. The study of these four needs will help you understand the whole procedure of managing your life much clearer. It is possible to adapt these principles to your personal social, religious or cultural background.

If you are trying to deal with all the aspects involved in managing your life it could be daunting, and you might not be able to begin meditating. The fact that there are only four areas you must focus on may provide ease.

Examining and Regulating the Four Urges

You are aware of the four desires however there are two aspects to managing the urges:

* You can observe the actions of these impulses and their relationship to the four functions of the mind buddhi ahamkara, Chitta, and manas. This means that you must be aware of your thoughts, words and actions.

* It controlled these desires in ways which don't cause obstacles to your meditation. This means that you must to make wise decisions.

When students attempt to discern their influence and control the desires, it will be clear what the fountains of desire are where needs, expectations as well as desires, needs, and wants are able to spring forth.

You will be able to immediately recognize how these four factors can trigger emotional reactions, influence your thoughts, and inadvertently direct your actions and speech. The unconscious impressions and tendencies which have been hidden in our unconscious will be made known when we meditate.

The two elements of observation and regulation identical to the question "Which is more important which is the egg or the chicken?" The truth is both of them always recycle in the opposite direction. Thus, there is always the cycle of chicken, egg and egg, as well as chicken and so on. Regulations and observations could be recycled into observation, regulation and observation. observation, etc.

A certain degree of regulation may provide a better setting for observation. Being able to see things more clearly will result in a greater control capability by making clear choices and having more determination.

It will gradually transform into a stunning dance of control and observation, which will eventually lead you to the peace of mind that is taught. Then you will be able to develop an even deeper meditation.

When you are progressing through your meditations, it is important to keep in mind that observation and regulation have a connection, similar to how the left and right foot while walking. You've been kind and kind to yourself as you were moving ahead.

Food

The recommended amount of water you should drink will differ according to the person you are talking to, however, at a minimum, you should take eight glasses of water each daily. That means that you should consume around two quarts of water a each day. Double this amount can help to ensure your body is clean. The most effective way to determine whether you're getting enough fluids is to look at the color of your urine. Every morning when you get up you will notice that your urine is likely to be a little darker.

Color to eat. If you find that your urine is a different hue in the course of the day, then you're drinking too much water. Your urine should have pale yellow in color.

Vitamins

There are many views on taking vitamins. I'm not going to start a discussion over it. While you're eating healthy and believe you're receiving all the vitamins and minerals you require from your diet there could be an "hole" that isn't being filled with nutritional intake. There could be a mineral or vitamin you've not been getting in your diet.

One approach to address it is taking multivitamins each day. It is possible to try this for a brief period and observe whether you feel better. If you notice changes, you could have discovered an "hole" within your food regimen. You can look at your diet to discover the deficiencies and if you find it, you can modify your intake of vitamins to address the deficit or continue to take your multivitamin. It is just important to take note of the fact that there may be an "hole" within your diet and handle this issue to your best abilities.

Conclusion

Pranayama is an antiquated art that is practiced without belief in God or the supernatural. You don't have to start practicing yoga. It has a variety of amazing health claims and, although some of them can hold up to scrutiny by scientists however, many others aren't able to prove themselves.

The increasing popularity of this technique is proof of its fact it's far from simply a trend. As with those who've tried it before increasing numbers of people are beginning to realize the benefits of this technique. This is great because it encourages people in the scientific community to study at it more deeply and who is to say what other claims about health may be proved to be true in the near future?

Breath is life in all likelihood, but as with everything it is important to approach pranayama with a certain amount of care. The benefits of pranayama could also harm and, as the old authors and doctors of today have proven -- the things that heal can also cause harm.

Adham pranayama is the most secure practice that is available. All of us begin pranayama at a young age, and as toddlers at the very least.

As puberty approaches, we begin to forget. Begin pranayama with adham and then observe the way you feel. Based on your results and your doctor's guidance, you are able to continue with the rest of the practice.